HEALTHY MOTHER, HEALTHY BABY

HEALTHY MOTHER, HEALTHY BABY

THE COMPLETE GUIDE
FOR NEW MOTHERS

Aliza A. Lifshitz, M.D.
La Doctora Aliza

RUTLEDGE HILL PRESS®
Nashville, Tennessee

A Division of Thomas Nelson Publishers
www.ThomasNelson.com

Published by Rutledge Hill Press, a Division of Thomas Nelson, Inc., P.O. Box 141000, Nashville, Tennessee 37214.

Rutledge Hill Press books may be purchased in bulk for educational, business, fundraising, or sales promotional use. For information, please e-mail SpecialMarkets@ThomasNelson.com.

Originally published in 1999 by Avon Books, and in 2002 by HarperCollins Publishers.

Illustrations by Aida T. Magdaluyo.

Jacket photography by Bob D'Amico.

Library of Congress Cataloging-in-Publication Data

Lifshitz, Aliza A.
[Mamá sana, bebé sano. English]
    Healthy mother, healthy baby : the complete guide for new mothers / Aliza A. Lifshitz.
        p. cm.
Includes bibliographical references and index.
    ISBN-13: 978-1-4016-0298-7 (trade paper)
    ISBN-10: 1-4016-0298-3 (trade paper)
    1. Pregnancy. 2. Prenatal care. I. Title.
RG525.L54313 2006
618.2—dc22
                                                                2006014594

Printed in the United States of America

06 07 08 09 10 — 5 4 3 2 1

Making the decision to have a child—it's momentous. It is to decide forever to have your heart go walking around outside your body.

—ELIZABETH STONE

CONTENTS

ACKNOWLEDGMENTS

In the years I have spent practicing medicine and striving to educate the public through the media, I have learned an important lesson—the best teachers are those most willing to learn from their students. And so, to my students (my patients), for all the lessons I have learned from you, my heartfelt thanks. My gratitude to you who have shared with me your time and thoughts, your questions and concerns. And to my own teachers and mentors, both in Mexico and in the United States, I will always be indebted.

I am very grateful to my husband, Carl, my friend, for his patience, his love, his support, and his willingness to read the manuscript and offer his suggestions in both languages.

My profound appreciation to Jessica Wainright, more than a literary agent, an enthusiastic friend whose encouragement, energy, and support for the book were a large part of making it happen, and to Omar Amador, for his assistance as my collaborator and researcher. His professionalism and wit made writing this book a wonderful experience.

I would like to thank Lidia Rubinstein, M.D., a friend and colleague who was willing to review and give me her input on the book. To my beloved sister Vivian Lombrozo, thank you for helping me to review the final manuscript. My thanks also to Cristina Saralegui, Maria Elena Salinas, Myrka Dellanos, and all the celebrities who were willing to share their experiences during pregnancy with us.

Special thanks to Luis and Rosita Nogales for their friendship and always thoughtful, thorough, and valuable advice.

Thanks to Maite and Bob D'Amico, the artists who helped me with the cover photograph.

A debt of gratitude is due to Alejandro Gil, M.D., who has graciously covered my practice, far too often, so that I could devote time to writing.

I also wish to thank all the health advocates who fight for patients and for access to care for everyone. I am grateful to the friends and colleagues whom I've had the pleasure of meeting through medical organizations and other institutions and from whom I've learned so much.

This book would not have happened without the support of my loyal staff, Maria Amador and Maria (Maru) Coronado. They help care for my patients, always with a smile.

Last, but not least, I want to thank my exceptional family and my friends (they know who they are) for the love and support they've always given me. And to my parents without whom I would not be here. Thanks to their love, their guidance, their example, and their kindness, I've become who I am. Without them, nothing would have been possible.

INTRODUCTION

Ask any mother on the planet about the happiest moments in her life, and she'll immediately tell you about when she first held her baby in her arms.

There's no doubt that feminism, despite all it has accomplished in society and the workplace, hasn't found a substitute—for the majority of women—for that profound deep inner fulfillment that comes, by nature, from our chief, exclusive, and most intense occupation: carrying a new being in our womb and giving it life.

The birth of a baby is the culmination of a period full of special precautions, visits to the doctor, changes in diet and physical exercise, and increasing anxiety on the part of the future mother and the rest of her family as the time of birth approaches.

Nonetheless, although there are hundreds of universities in which women can prepare themselves to become lawyers, engineers, teachers, physicians, or businesswomen, there isn't a single institution in the world that teaches them the challenging career of being a mother. You can only learn about motherhood in the "school of life." The course doesn't end in nine months. That is only the elementary phase. This career lasts a lifetime.

In past years, women faced the moment of giving birth armed with information they received from their own mothers, their grandmothers, and other close relatives. The wisdom of relatives and friends was not always correct, and many myths still survive. In those days, pregnancy was considered to be almost an illness and not what it really is: a natural state for a woman's body to undergo as it changes throughout a nine-month period. Thus, in many instances pregnant women—especially first timers—have regarded the onset of the symptoms of delivery with terror, not knowing what they could do for themselves to facilitate and advance the process, and thinking that everything lay in the doctor's hands.

I originally wrote this book to put the power and the knowledge back into the prospective mother's hands.

Even though children are still made the "old-fashioned way" and technology has not changed a lot since the first edition of this book seven years ago, there are a few things we have learned and an increase in the number of services available to new parents. This book reflects these changes and includes an up-to-date list of resources.

It is true that the birth of a baby changes everybody around him: parents, grandparents, sisters and brothers, and extended families, but what changes the most is the baby himself. It is up to us to give him the best opportunity to arrive in this world healthy and loved. I believe that the responsibility of new parents begins long before they hold their baby in their arms. For women, preparing for pregnancy really begins when they become teenagers and are able to conceive. If you think about it, what she eats, whether or not she smokes or drinks, who she chooses as a sexual partner, and whether or not she gets a sexually transmitted disease will all have an impact on her ability to get pregnant. So much so that the March of Dimes, an organization devoted to the prevention of birth defects, recommends that all women of childbearing age take a daily supplement of folic acid. If a woman is not planning a pregnancy and starts taking it when she finds out that she is pregnant, she may have lost an opportunity. This book helps future mothers and their partners review their options and make informed decisions. This book can help any couple, whether they are thinking of becoming parents in the future or whether they are already involved in the process of childbearing, since the information they receive will allow them to enjoy the journey more and to participate fully.

THE HISPANIC MOTHER

We are all aware of the difficulties a family encounters when it emigrates from its native country. Hispanics who come to this country have to learn a new language to advance economically. They also have to adapt to new customs and to a lifestyle that's a lot faster than those in their native countries.

A woman who, in many instances, has had a life limited to her duties as a homemaker suddenly has to learn a trade or profession and find a job in order to contribute to the family finances. And, on top of that, if she decides to have a child, she no longer has the nearby support of the relatives who stayed behind.

For people of other cultures, this wouldn't be so important. But it is a genuine problem for Hispanic women who come from a culture in which the nuclear family—with the mother at the center—is the basic support system.

So it's easy to conclude that, at this time—along with the joy of knowing she will soon be a mother—she may fear that she won't be able to face the event alone.

When a Hispanic woman can count on the company and support of her mother or another close relative, she will most likely face a confrontation between the customs of her native country and those of the United States' modern society. In her home country, if that older relative had more than four children, she never left her house to give birth because she didn't think it was necessary. That older relative might consider it ridiculous for a future mother to visit a specialist regularly and to decide to give birth in a hospital.

It would not be unusual for an older relative to relate beliefs and superstitions about pregnancy that have no basis in scientific fact but that are handed down from generation to generation in Hispanic countries. For example, some believe that if a pregnant woman puts her hand on her belly during a lunar eclipse, her child will be born with a dark spot on whichever part of the body she touched. Others are convinced that you can predict the sex of the baby by having a pregnant woman with her eyes closed sit on a chair under which a pair of scissors and a knife have been placed. If the mother sits on the knife, she will have a boy. If she sits on the scissors, she will have a girl. Still others believe that if a pregnant woman doesn't satisfy a craving, her baby will be born with its mouth open. Or that, if her belly is rounded, she'll give birth to a girl, while if it's pointed, she'll have a boy. And these stories go on.

Though there may be wisdom in some popular beliefs, the most sensible thing is to not set too much store by them. Try to avoid discussing them with people who believe in them—the only thing you'll get is an argument, and they'll probably never change their minds anyway. It's better just to enjoy their love and attention, which truly are sincere and well-intentioned.

In any case, the pregnant woman has a right to decide whether or not she wants to work with her doctor in order to have a healthy baby. Above all, she has the right to be informed of all the risks of her pregnancy and of the ways she should respond in case there is a problem. And, of course, if she has her mother or grandmother by her side, she'll have even more care and understanding during the time she'll need it most.

IGNORANCE IS AT THE ROOT OF FEAR

During the years I've been in practice, I've treated countless pregnant women. Many were my patients before they became pregnant. What I've observed is that all of them express apprehension once the birth of their child draws near.

It's perfectly normal to feel fear and anxiety as that moment approaches, but those feelings can be overcome if the woman knows what is going on inside of her and how her baby is developing.

Imagine that you were teaching a child to swim. If you tossed him, without prior warning, into deep ocean water, the only thing you'd accomplish would be to convince him never to want to go back to the beach, much less ever to learn to swim a stroke. The result is different if, while you're in the shallow end of a pool or at the water's edge, you first teach him the movements he has to perform. With more knowledge and information, he is less afraid about taking a plunge into the ocean.

Something similar was the norm just a few years ago, when women arrived at their deliveries without knowing what was going to happen to them or what they had to do to avoid suffering. It was much more traumatic than a plunge into ice-cold water. The brave ones who repeated the experience had to learn along the way because "that was a woman's destiny," and that's "why women were brought into the world."

In some cases, a pregnant woman's fears stem from the fact that, ever since childhood (mostly from listening to women from earlier generations), she has been unconsciously indoctrinated. If her mother had a difficult birth, she probably told her daughter about that traumatic experience, causing her daughter to fear that the same thing will happen to her. There is no reason for that fear, since no pregnancy is like any other, not even when it concerns the same woman.

The media also influences the fears of first-time mothers. If births were really like the ones on the "telenovelas," surely the human race would've died out many years ago! No woman can help give birth to her child by screaming. At the moment of birth, she needs all of her lung capacity in order to push and keep the baby oxygenated. This is totally impossible to do if you are screaming at the top of your lungs like the soap opera heroines we see giving birth on television. You shouldn't let yourself be influenced by these images. They are fiction.

The most important thing for the mother-to-be is to insist on getting all the information she can on her state, discarding any false modesty and asking her doctor everything she wants to know, without being afraid of appearing ignorant. The more she trusts her doctor, the more effective their collaboration. And that's the best prescription for a healthy birth.

PAPÁ HAS A RIGHT TO KNOW

Almost always, except for single mothers or couples who for some reason have to live apart, the future father is the family member who is closest to the pregnant woman. This is why there is no one better able to help her through this difficult stage. But good intentions aren't enough. It's hard for a man to help his wife during her pregnancy if he isn't informed.

Many men are discouraged to see that their wife is sad, or in a bad mood, or rejects certain foods while waking him up at dawn asking for others. Sometimes she doesn't want to be touched, and other times she is surprisingly insistent that she be made love to. Some men react by remaining distant because they don't know how to cope with these situations. In doing so, however, they deny their wives the care and affection they need so much.

For this reason, this book is also dedicated to them. Reading it, preferably along with the mother-to-be, will give the future father the knowledge and confidence he needs to be a collaborator in the prenatal development of his child, even though he's not carrying the baby in his womb. Following his wife's pregnancy step-by-step will help him enjoy his child even before she is born.

Few things unite a couple more than when a father places his hand or his head on his partner's belly in order to feel or hear the baby's kicks. Or when he talks to his child and sings to her softly during the last few months. Or his awareness that the baby is listening to him and learning to recognize his voice.

At the same time, these activities will help the new father get excited about attending the birth, give his partner moral support, and enjoy the unique privilege of seeing his child be born.

TEENAGE PREGNANCY

Although teenage pregnancy is not recommended because it might lead to miscarriages, premature births, low-weight babies, and mothers who are ill-prepared or unwilling to raise a child, it is something that happens frequently. If birth is a subject that invites questions, fears, and doubts in adult women, imagine what it is like for teenagers or very young adults! Many times the pregnant teenager hasn't even completed high school and is ignorant about anatomy and the way the body functions. In other cases, girls may know what they've learned in school, yet be surprised to learn that everything the biology professor taught them is about to happen to them!

Once a pregnancy is confirmed, the young girl must decide whether to follow her doctor's advice to the letter in order to avoid any complications that may arise. She must realize that, from this moment on, she will be responsible for the life that is growing in her womb, resulting in her having to care for two.

The most important part of this care is her diet. Many teenagers like nothing better than tacos, hamburgers, and pizza, which are undisputably delicious (once in a while). But they won't give the future mother the nutrients her baby needs in order to be born healthy.

The pages of this book can serve as a guide for the young mother on changing her dietary habits and eating a balanced diet rich in vitamins and minerals so that her baby will develop normally. In addition, she can correct any weight problems she may have that might not only affect the baby but make the birth process more difficult.

THE MATURE MOTHER

The opposite case is the mature woman who has waited many years to have a baby. Today it is quite normal to run into successful professional women who have put off the joy of being mothers until they have accomplished the goals they have set for their careers. This is admirable. But mature women have their own special health concerns and need information just as much as very young women.

The majority of these professional women want to continue working as long as their pregnancy allows. This leaves them little time to do extensive reading and to get information on all aspects of pregnancy and birthing. They will find this book particularly useful because of its accessible format.

THE GOAL OF THIS BOOK

There are many books in English regarding pregnancy and birth. But there are few in Spanish and no guide for the Hispanic woman. This book is addressed specifically to the Hispanic woman and is available in English and Spanish.

My objective is not to offer an overly extensive and detailed scientific documentation of this subject, but to create a book that women will find useful and accessible and friendly. I've also decided not to deal with subjects such as alternative medicine and certain types of births that are only performed occasionally, such as seated delivery or birth in water.

I address the basic aspects of pregnancy and the risks it can pose. I want pregnant women to know that, in their condition, it's normal to feel fear and anxiety. And I want each of them to understand that the more information she has about her pregnancy, the more confidence and control she will have during the difficult moments that may arise.

A large part of the success of the pregnancy depends on the woman knowing what's going on and how she should cope with certain situations. And above all, the woman should know that pregnancy is not an illness; it's a condition experienced by a healthy woman that requires special care.

Throughout the entire book, the mother-to-be will find text boxes with simple instructions, facts, suggestions, and comments on different subjects related to pregnancy. These range from suggestions on names for boys and girls to telephone numbers and addresses of help centers, unforgettable quotations on motherhood, recent medical studies on the health of mother and child, and statistics on pregnancy risks, among other things.

In *Healthy Mother, Healthy Baby,* you will also hear from several Hispanic mothers from the worlds of music and television who haven't forgotten how they felt during the days when they were about to bring their children into the world. These celebrities offer useful hints to future mothers, which are found only in this book, based on their own experiences during pregnancy.

In order for the reader to better understand *Healthy Mother, Healthy Baby,* I have included a glossary defining the words that relate to pregnancy and birth, words that the pregnant woman will encounter during her nine-month term or at the time of birth.

I wrote this book in a way that gives the reader a choice. He or she can read it from beginning to end, read each month as the pregnancy progresses, just look for answers to questions she may have, use it to better understand certain terms in English and/or Spanish, or look for services that may be available in specific areas.

In our Hispanic culture, pregnant women have always had—in addition to the professional advice of doctors—the comfort and experience of a relative or friend at home in whom they could confide. *Healthy Mother, Healthy Baby* hopes to become that friendly voice, which, through user-friendly informative text, will show you what to do and what to expect during these nine months, in the affectionate tone the Hispanic family has traditionally expected from their family doctor. Someone who is a friend more than a physician.

There is no substitute for a pregnant woman's relationship with her doctor. This book has absolutely no intention of replacing the obstetrician. He or she will be in charge of providing specific information not found in this book. Childbirth is the most natural and yet the most awesome of experiences. It's one of life's most fascinating adventures. The goal of this book is to make pregnancy and delivery less mysterious and frightening, without taking away its "magic." I hope you will enjoy it and find it helpful.

—ALIZA A. LIFSHITZ, M.D.

Chapter 1

FIRST THINGS FIRST

The birth of a baby is magical. It never ceases to amaze me. At the first delivery I ever witnessed as a medical student, I was so intensely moved that I cried longer and harder than the mother who had just given birth. Each person evolves following the fertilization of an egg, so minute that it can't be seen without the help of a microscope, by an even smaller sperm. When they join together, they become an embryo, which is like a small orb that encapsules all the necessary information with which to create an autonomous human being. It contains all it needs in order to determine the different organs that must be made, the place they must occupy within the body and their function, information about the color of the eyes and hair, as well as the fact that, at nine months, the development within the mother will cease, only to be continued independently after birth. Birth is the glorious moment when this little being becomes a new individual who breathes, feels, eats, cries, smiles, and begins to relate with the environment.

Ideally, you hope your pregnancy and delivery will be perfect, especially considering all the technology presently available. But there are no guarantees. There are certain things that can be done, though, that may help prevent problems or detect them at an early stage. The mother's health and her gynecological and medical background, as well as her family's, play an important role.

IF YOU ARE THINKING ABOUT GETTING PREGNANT

Your pregnancy should be a very special experience that, ideally, you will remember with love. If you take care of yourself and are prepared before becoming pregnant, your chances of having that kind of experience are excellent. Your physical health and your nutrition help determine whether your pregnancy is easy or more difficult. Though you may feel well, have your doctor examine you before you become pregnant. If you have any condition such as diabetes, hypertension, hypothyroidism, asthma, etc., see your doctor and make sure that it's under control and that you are taking the proper medication. This will increase your chances of becoming pregnant and of helping your baby develop and grow under the best circumstances.

BEFORE GETTING PREGNANT, CONSIDER THE FOLLOWING

- Begin an exercise program (if you are not already on one).
- Lose weight if you are overweight (expectant mothers should not be dieting).
- Take care of having any procedures you may require (such as X-rays recommended by your doctor for back pain or for dental work); you will not be able to do so once you are pregnant.
- Stop smoking and drinking alcoholic beverages. This is the best time to do so.
- Check with your doctor if you take vitamins, herbs, or other medication, regarding their effect on your baby should you become pregnant. He or she may recommend that you supplement your diet with vitamins.
- Make sure you are getting enough folic acid. One milligram a day at least three months before becoming pregnant helps prevent some birth defects.
- Talk with your doctor if you have not had German measles and have not had the vaccination; your doctor may want to run a blood test to find out whether you have the antibodies and/or give you a vaccination to prevent problems once you are pregnant.
- If you get the German measles vaccine, wait three months after the immunizations to get pregnant.

IF YOU THINK YOU ARE PREGNANT

As soon as you realize, or imagine, or think you may be pregnant, it is important to see your doctor. Even though there are several possible reasons for missing your period—including nervous tension, overwork, weight change, or excessive exercising—it is important to know whether you are pregnant. I have patients who say, "Well, I've already had one (or four) children without any problems. I know I have to take my prenatal vitamins and eat well and not gain too much weight.... Why should I see the doctor now? I'll wait." My answer is, *don't wait*. Each pregnancy is different and requires medical supervision in order to detect whether there is any problem that may not have been present earlier. Seeing your doctor early increases the chances that *this* pregnancy will be an uncomplicated one.

SYMPTOMS THAT MIGHT SUGGEST PREGNANCY

- Absence of a menstrual period
- A very light menstrual period
- A change in the size of your breasts, increased sensitivity, or slight discomfort. It is possible that you may feel discomfort, such as the kind some women experience a few days prior to menstruation, which then disappears when menstruation begins. If you are pregnant, the discomfort may continue for several weeks and be accompanied by a tingling sensation in the nipples and visible increase in their size. This is due to the mammary glands, which are preparing to produce the milk that will feed your baby.
- Nausea due to increased hormonal production
- An increase in the frequency of urination. The uterus is growing and presses on the bladder. This symptom disappears in the third month and reappears in the last trimester of the pregnancy, when the baby's weight increases dramatically.
- Cravings and food preferences. Were you among those who believed cravings were "tall tales" told by pregnant women? You may notice it happening to you. In any case, eating a little more of the foods you crave will not harm you, as long as you maintain a balanced diet.
- Fatigue

- Slight increase in vaginal secretions. This can be a normal symptom during pregnancy, due to the increase of hormones. A laboratory exam by your doctor will rule out an infection.
- Increased saliva production in the initial months

TESTS TO CONFIRM YOUR PREGNANCY

All pregnancy tests are based on the presence of the hormone known as human chorionic gonadotropin (HCG). The placenta produces this hormone, and it may be detected in female urine or blood.

HOME TESTING

Pharmacies sell test kits over the counter that require only a urine sample. Among them are "First Response," "EPT," "Clearblue Easy Digital," "Fact Plus Select," and "Answer One-Step." Some include instructions in Spanish. They are excellent for women who don't have the patience to see a doctor in order to find out if they are pregnant. The cost varies between $10 and $23. They do not require a prescription. Though they are not infallible, they are more precise when used correctly. They are considered quick and practical initial home tests. The final diagnosis should be determined by a medical examination.

All home tests are more precise when the instructions are followed carefully and when the menstrual period is at least two weeks late. If the result is negative, repeat the test a week later. If the second result also proves negative, the chances of a pregnancy are doubtful. However, even though the result from a home pregnancy test is negative, you should see your doctor immediately after missing a second menstrual period. It could be the sign of some other problem.

There are circumstances when the results are positive although there is no pregnancy, and vice versa.

Some of the causes of a *false positive* result (in other words, the woman is not pregnant, but the test results are positive) are:

- The woman has recently used marijuana, methadone, or certain medications, such as methyldopa (known as Aldomet), which is prescribed in the treatment of hypertension.
- The woman has a type of cancer known as hydatidiform mole.

Some of the causes of a *false negative* result (in other words, the woman is pregnant, but the test results are negative) are:

- The urine is very diluted.
- The test is not performed within a relatively short time after the urine sample is taken.
- The container holding the sample is contaminated or dirty.
- The test is carried out too early in the pregnancy.

LABORATORY TESTS

As I indicated earlier, lab tests are based on the presence of human chorionic gonadotropin in the urine or blood that your doctor sends to a laboratory.

Besides confirming the pregnancy with a urine or blood sample, your doctor may detect certain changes—such as an increase in the size of the womb—from a pelvic examination. A pelvic examination diagnosis is more accurate after eight weeks of pregnancy. Naturally, this examination does not affect the baby.

The blood test may be qualitative, meaning it tells whether there is a pregnancy, or it may be quantitative. Quantitative means that it provides your doctor with a number. Along with the date of your last period, this number may help the doctor determine the date of delivery. The quantity of human chorionic gonadotropin hormone increases as the pregnancy advances. Its quantity may be used to evaluate growth and the normal progress of the pregnancy.

In the event of an ectopic pregnancy (in other words, a pregnancy where the baby is not growing inside the womb), the result of the pregnancy test will be positive. But, usually, these pregnancies do not reach term and they may endanger the mother's life. **For this reason, even if you feel well, if your home test result is positive, you must see your doctor as soon as possible.**

MYTH

If the mother's belly is pointed, it's a boy; if it's round, it's a girl. The shape of the mother's belly depends on several factors: how strong her abdominal muscles are, the position of the baby, whether there are one or more babies, her posture when standing, the shape and size of her pelvis, etc. First timers generally tend to have stronger muscles and smaller bellies, and the baby is usually carried higher up. None of what I have said has anything to do with the baby's gender. Any accurate prediction is mere coincidence.

YOUR OBSTETRICIAN

If you were to have a baby, you would probably not take him to just any pediatrician, right? Well, the same applies to choosing the doctor who will monitor your pregnancy. The fact is, the obstetrician will be your baby's doctor . . . until it is born.

- He or she must be a professional with a degree in medicine and must have specialized in obstetrics and gynecology.
- Ideally your doctor should be someone who is recommended by a relative or friend who has been her patient, or who is recommended by another doctor you trust.
- You must trust the doctor enough to share all of your concerns regarding your pregnancy, and he or she must be comfortable speaking your own language.
- It is also important to ask who would deliver the baby in the event your doctor were not on call that day.
- Ideally, your doctor will be associated with the hospital where you wish to deliver your baby.

CURANDERISMO

Curanderismo is the art practiced by *curanderos*, those who employ herbs, spiritualism, and/or religious subjects for the purpose of healing. This tradition has been practiced for hundreds, or even thousands, of years. It was begun by the Mayas and the Aztecs in pre-Columbian Mexico. It is an art that, even today, has loyal followers, with testimonials given by people who say they have been healed from all kinds of known diseases, ranging from physical to mental, in both children and adults. In some rural areas there are people who have never been to a doctor, yet claim the *curandero* has cured them of all their "ailments." *Curanderos* may occasionally deliver babies, but they are not legally licensed to do so. Relying on such a practitioner is potentially dangerous to your baby's health, and to your own.

VISITING THE DOCTOR

There will always be those who will tell you that you visit the doctor too often and that it is not necessary because you are a healthy woman. They will give you an example of a mother who had healthy children with no medical assistance at all. You should simply reply that, thanks to pregnancy supervision, complications have been greatly reduced, both for mothers and their babies. Your chances of having a healthy baby and of minimizing maternity risks are directly linked to early medical prenatal care.

YOUR FIRST VISIT TO THE DOCTOR

Ideally, this should happen as soon as you suspect you might be pregnant. It is useful to make a note of the date when your last menstrual period began. Avoid douches before your visit, as this could eliminate certain significant secretions important to your gynecological examination. The answers you give your doctor should be as precise as possible. Feel free to ask any and all questions that will clear up any doubts you may have.

What you should expect from your first visit:
- Confirmation that you are pregnant, if you are
- Approximate date of delivery, calculated by using the date of your last period
- Understand the frequency of your future medical examinations
- Be aware of the signs or symptoms that may alert you to call your doctor or to go to an emergency room or to the hospital
- Learn recommendations on diet, exercise, and vitamins

What type of medical attention you will receive on this first visit:

You will be asked general questions about your health, the health of the baby's father, and the health of your parents and the father's parents.

DISCLOSING INFORMATION TO YOUR DOCTOR

Do not hide information from the doctor concerning previous illnesses, possible abortions or pregnancies, relatives who may suffer from hereditary diseases, or any other subject—no matter how embarrassing or private it seems. Even though you may not feel comfortable discussing certain things, it is essential to your pregnancy that your doctor be aware of EVERYTHING that may affect your health and your baby's health. If the obstetrician does not have all the necessary information, he or she may not be able to give you the best medical attention.

What makes up your medical history:

Your doctor will take your medical history. The information needed concerns your health, the health of your family, and whether you have had previous pregnancies. It is important that you answer honestly and offer as much information as possible. This information is confidential. You should mention whether you are taking any medication (even those that do not require prescriptions, e.g., aspirin), whether you are suffering from a medical problem (such as diabetes, high blood pressure, or asthma), if you have allergies, if you have received any blood transfusions, whether you've had any surgery or previous infections (such as hepatitis), if you have had German measles or have been vaccinated against it, or if you smoke, drink alcoholic beverages, or have used drugs.

Family history is important in order to determine whether there is any possibility of a hereditary disease. Sometimes, if you have had a child with a medical problem, certain tests are recommended in subsequent pregnancies. A consultation with a genetics specialist (someone who deals with hereditary diseases) may be in order.

What makes up your gynecological-obstetrical history:

The information on your gynecological and obstetrical *history* is as important to your doctor as any information resulting from each of your visits concerning the evolution of your pregnancy.

It is important that your doctor be well informed about any problem or previous condition because, though these circumstances may bear no immediate relation to this pregnancy, they will help your doctor know more about your body and how it has functioned and responded in the past.

Before your visit, make a list of the health problems you have had so you don't forget any of them. Include everything, for example, abortions (miscarriage or induced), previous pregnancies, surgeries, sexually transmitted diseases, etc.

Do not censor your information for moral reasons based on what the doctor may think of previous pregnancies, previous infections, etc. Your doctor needs this information in order to make a thorough evaluation and therefore prevent problems. He or she is not there to pass judgment on you or on your past.

If you have had other pregnancies, it will be important to mention the baby's (or babies') weight at birth, how long labor lasted, whether delivery was vaginal or by cesarean section, whether anesthesia was administered and whether there were any complications, for example, premature delivery (before the nine-month term), high blood pressure or diabetes during pregnancy or delivery, infections, bleeding, or any complications concerning breast-feeding.

What the physical examination will evaluate:

- Your height and weight
- Your blood pressure
- Your overall health from head to toe, listening to your heart and lungs, and a breast, abdominal, and pelvic examination

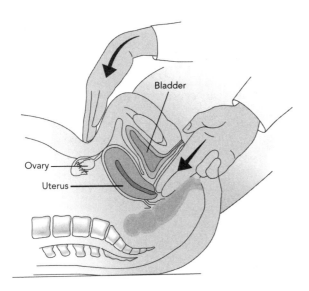

Pelvic exam

With the woman lying on her back with her legs bent, the obstetrician inserts two fingers in the vagina and places his or her hand on the patient's abdomen to palpate the womb and the ovaries.

What the blood and urine tests and ultrasound look for:

You will be given a battery of tests. Among them are the following:

- A test to determine your blood type and Rh factor
- A test to determine the level of hemoglobin in your blood, to rule out anemia
- A test to detect the presence of antibodies against German measles (if you have not been vaccinated, have not had the disease, or you don't know whether you have)
- A test for syphilis and other sexually transmitted diseases
- A test for hepatitis antibodies
- A Pap smear, if you have not had one in the last year (to rule out the presence of cancer cells in the neck of the womb or cervix)
- A test for the HIV/AIDS virus
- A urine sample to test for sugar and protein; this may suggest diabetes, kidney trouble, or infections

- If you are over thirty-five, or there is a family history or possible susceptibility to certain diseases, your doctor might recommend certain special examinations (genetic) and, later on, an examination of the fluid that surrounds the fetus in the womb (amniotic fluid), known as amniocentesis.
- An ultrasound to determine if the pregnancy is inside the uterus, whether the fetus has heartbeats already, and whether the size coincides with the dates of pregnancy (see Chapter 3)

Several of these tests will be repeated during the course of the pregnancy.

WHAT ELSE IS IMPORTANT ON THIS FIRST VISIT?

It is important that you ask all the questions necessary to address any doubts you may have about your pregnancy. Express your fears and expectations openly and without hesitation. The more information you have, the easier your pregnancy will be. This will probably be your longest visit.

SUBSEQUENT VISITS

The frequency of the medical examinations varies from woman to woman, but generally you should expect the following:

If you do not have other medical problems and you feel well, your doctor will see you every four to six weeks during the first seven months of the pregnancy. Starting with the eighth month (or thirty-two weeks), you will be seen every two weeks. In the final month, your visits will be on a weekly basis. Make sure you discuss any symptoms you have and ask any questions regarding doubts you may have. If necessary, write them down and take them with you.

At each visit, your doctor will check your weight and blood pressure, examine the size of your womb, and, as the pregnancy advances, check the size and position of the baby as well as his heartbeat. A urine sample will also be taken to test for the presence of sugar and protein.

At sixteen weeks, a blood test known as alpha-fetoprotein will be routinely performed to determine any abnormalities in the development of the baby's nervous system. At thirty weeks, a test will check the level of sugar in the blood to rule out gestational diabetes (see Chapter 2) and a blood cell count will rule out anemia (lowering of red blood cell count).

Do not assume that, because you are feeling well, you can monitor your pregnancy on your own. Not going to the doctor, though you feel healthy over several months, endangers your health and your baby's health.

The ideal number of visits to the doctor during the nine months of pregnancy is twelve to thirteen. Do not miss any of these. During the final month, do not miss your weekly appointments—right up to the moment of delivery.

In case you have other medical problems such as asthma, hypertension, diabetes, heart disease, or a complication during the pregnancy, your doctor will indicate the frequency of visits and whether further tests are required.

WHEN YOU SHOULD CALL YOUR DOCTOR

There are certain signs or symptoms that could arise during the pregnancy and that must be immediately communicated to your doctor, because they could be important. Among them are:

Vaginal bleeding. Although it is very common during the first three months of the pregnancy, it could also signal the threat of a miscarriage. Obviously the amount of bleeding, its duration, and whether it is accompanied by pain are very important details.

Abdominal pain. Light discomfort in the abdomen due to the baby's growth within the womb, or even minor contraction sensations when the baby moves, are common. However, if the pain is severe or persists, notify your doctor.

Frequent vomiting. Nausea and vomiting, especially in the first three months of the pregnancy, are very common. But if they persist and are severe, notify your doctor.

Fever. This is the same as when you are not pregnant. If you are running an elevated temperature, it generally means there is an infection. This could be as simple as the flu, but it could also be due to an infection in the urinary tract or reproductive organs, which may require treatment with antibiotics.

Swelling of face, hands, and/or feet. When the swelling, which is due to water retention, is severe or increases, especially during the final months of the pregnancy, it is important to notify your doctor. It could be an early signal of eclampsia or toxemia (a complication we will discuss later in Chapter 3).

Blurred vision. If you notice blurred vision, notify your doctor. This could also signal eclampsia. If you are diabetic, it could mean your sugar levels are out of control.

Severe and persistent headaches. Although frequently due to sinus congestion, this could also mean retention of fluids and eclampsia.

Vaginal discharge. It is normal for vaginal discharge to increase during pregnancy, but it is not normal for the discharge to be accompanied by other symptoms (such as burning, itching, etc.). If you detect an excessive amount of discharge, it could also mean that your water has broken (in other words, the amniotic fluid that surrounds the baby), in which case you must notify your doctor immediately.

Excessive thirst. This could be due to an increase in sugar levels in the blood (possible diabetes).

Several studies indicate that pregnant women who visit their doctor often deliver healthier babies and suffer fewer complications. However, in addition to your appointments, you must notify your doctor of any discomfort or doubts you may have. There are problems that, even though they seem harmless initially, could develop into serious complications.

LAY MIDWIVES (UNLICENSED)

Midwives (*parteras*) have played an important role, especially among Hispanics of lower socioeconomic Mexican descent. Historically, as with *curanderos*, most of them have no formal education. Not only do they assist in home delivery, but frequently their role within the community is as a member of the extended family, as are *curanderos* and wet nurses. *Parteras* are not doctors and are not trained to deal with medical issues.

If you choose to use a midwife, make sure that she is a certified nurse-midwife (CNM) or a certified midwife (CM). Certified midwives are trained and know to call a physician or refer to a hospital in case of an emergency. Lay midwives (*parteras no certificadas*) do not have the training to provide you and your baby with optimal care. If you are over the age of thirty-five or have a high-risk pregnancy, a midwife, even if she is certified, is not an option.

CERTIFIED NURSE-MIDWIVES

Certified nurse-midwives are medical professionals trained to care for women with low-risk pregnancies and to attend uncomplicated deliveries.

CALCULATING THE DUE DATE

Although we generally speak of the "nine months" of pregnancy, the actual length of the pregnancy is ten days longer. That is why gynecologists talk of "weeks" thirty-six to forty rather than months, as this is a more accurate measurement. Even more exact is the day count: 280. You will notice that, within a few weeks, you will be counting weeks as well as months.

Nobody can predict your delivery date precisely. There are certain general guidelines used to obtain an approximate date. These are based on women with a regular twenty-eight-day menstrual cycle. It is very simple, and even though your doctor will calculate it during your first visit, you may, if you wish, do it before. There are two ways of doing it:

CALCULATING THE DUE DATE

■ Beginning on the first day of your last period, add seven days and subtract three months. For example, if the first day of your last period was April 12, add seven days, which is April 19. Subtract three months from April 19 and your date will be January 19. That is the approximate date of your delivery.

-or-

■ Beginning with the first day of your last period, add 280 days.

In fact, the date calculation considered normal includes the two-week periods before and after. So, the best advice is to have your overnight bag ready fifteen days ahead of the calculated date. If more than two weeks past the estimated date go by, your doctor may recommend inducing delivery (in other words, administering an intravenous solution and/or breaking the water sac to induce the delivery) or performing a cesarean section, depending on your individual case. This is done because when the placenta gets old, it is no longer able to nourish the baby.

RIGHTS OF WORKING MOTHERS

It is estimated that, every year, more than one million working women in the United States become pregnant. Eighty-five percent of them work up until the last month. If you work you should do the following:

- Notify your employer of your pregnancy at the time that you wish to request your leave of absence (ideally during the third trimester).
- Check your company's regulations concerning pregnancy and those of the state where you reside, before you become pregnant.
- Advise your supervisors when you intend to return to work, allowing enough time to recover and to make adequate arrangements for the baby's care.
- Understand the law, which states that if you work for a company employing fifty or more workers, you are allowed up to twelve weeks of "maternity leave," without salary, and that, following that period, you may return to your job with the same full benefits as before.
- Be aware of the 1978 Pregnancy Discrimination Act, which states that pregnant women in companies of fifteen or more employees must be treated equally. Under this law, a pregnant woman must be given the same health, absenteeism, or disability benefits that any other employee would be given for medical reasons. These benefits include simpler labor tasks, alternating shifts, assurance of job recovery after delivery, accumulation of vacation days, etc.

YOUR WORK AND THE HEALTH OF
THE BABY YOU ARE EXPECTING

It is possible that the pressures pregnant women undergo at work could contribute to the incidence of premature births. According to Dr. Barbara Luke, from the Medical Center at the University of Michigan at Ann Arbor, "The number of premature births has increased due to the fact that the number of working women in the United States has doubled in the last thirty-five years." Standing for extended periods, excessive physical exertion, irregular working hours or extended hours on the job, fatigue, and work pressure may have contributed to a 20 percent increase in the number of premature births in the last decade. Dr. Luke goes on to suggest that this situation could be eased if pregnant women were allowed three preventive measures: reduced hours per week or per shift; reassigning of job activities so they are less exhausting; and access to maternity leave before the ninth month, especially in cases where the women have complications during their pregnancy.

HOW TO TAKE CARE OF YOURSELF AT WORK

- If you work sitting down, you should do a little walking every hour to activate circulation. Keep your feet up when you sit. Every so often, you should also do exercises to stretch your legs: for instance, extending and flexing your feet. Use a pillow in the small of your back and push your waist forward slightly when you feel too much pressure.
- If you work on your feet, take twenty-minute breaks or try to work sitting down. Working on your feet more than three hours a day increases the chances of a miscarriage. This is also true if you handle heavy or vibrating equipment, if you lift heavy objects, if you do repetitive movements, or if you are in an extremely noisy, hot, or cold environment.

- Whether sitting or standing, use comfortable shoes without heels and wear maternity hose or knee-highs. Dress in layers so that, should you feel warm, you can remove a layer.
- During your lunch break, find a quiet place where you can lie down.
- If you work for an industry using chemicals that may damage the development of the fetus, it is imperative that you act immediately and make inquiries with your doctor. Some chemicals may only cause certain discomfort during the pregnancy. However, others could provoke a miscarriage, a premature delivery, or birth defects.
- The first three months is the period of highest risk for exposure to toxic substances, especially the first six to eight weeks, which is when the baby's organs are being formed. Several substances are capable of crossing the placenta and reaching the fetus. Inquire at work if you are directly (or indirectly) exposed to one of the following substances:

Lead, nickel, cadmium, mercury, arsenic, dioxin

Detergents containing hexachlorophene

Solvents used in the making of plastics and rubber

- Ask if there is ionizing radiation (such as the kind caused by anesthetic gases) or areas where there is an abundance of dust, smoke, or gases such as carbon monoxide, among others; these may also be harmful. The same applies to excessive noise levels (particularly above 90 decibels) and cold or heat levels.
- Remember that if you work with children, you are more susceptible to common childhood infections such as measles, mumps, German measles, chicken pox, etc. Nowadays, there are several vaccinations against them. Hopefully you will have been vaccinated or have had the infection prior to planning your pregnancy. A specific blood test can determine whether you are immune by measuring the presence of antibodies against these infections. If you do not have the antibodies, it is important to avoid direct contact with children who may be infected, especially during the first three months of your pregnancy.

> ## YOUR LEGAL RIGHTS
>
> If you have any questions about your legal rights in the United States during pregnancy, you may call the Equal Employment Opportunity Commission at 1-800-669-4000 or go to www.eeoc.gov. Your questions will be answered in either English or Spanish.

THE ISSUE OF ABORTION AND RELIGION

Legalizing or banning abortion has been one of the most controversial subjects in modern society worldwide.

The Roman Catholic Church is firmly opposed to the practice of abortion, considering it a criminal act that goes against Divine will. However, at the same time, there are hair-raising statistics on women who, in areas where abortion is not legal (in the United States abortion *is* legal), have lost their lives as a consequence of abortions undertaken by unqualified people in an environment that lacks the necessary asepsis (cleanliness). That is why a woman facing the dilemma of whether to terminate her pregnancy must take several different perspectives into account, from both an ethical and a physical standpoint.

ETHICAL CONSIDERATIONS

Almost all religions consider inducing abortion a crime. The Catholic Church and the groups opposing abortion—many of them not connected to the Vatican—base their arguments mainly on the belief that what the woman carries inside her, from the very moment of conception, is a human being with life and that using abortion methods is equal to murder.

The advocates of legalizing abortion consider that abortion within the first three months of pregnancy is a personal option for a woman. She is, after all, responsible for the new life she will carry in her body during the nine months of the pregnancy and even after the baby is born. They defend the woman's right not to bring an unwanted child into the world, either under inappropriate living conditions or because it might be doomed to an early death due to a genetic deformity.

These groups argue that it is preferable to legalize abortion so that women making this choice have access to centers, with hygienic conditions that meet the necessary standards for surgical intervention, where the procedure is performed by qualified individuals.

According to this point of view, outlawing abortion encourages the practice of illegal abortions by unscrupulous people, in the absence of sufficient knowledge or sanitary conditions, causing irreparable damage . . . including the death of some of the women who fall into their hands.

HEALTH CONSIDERATIONS

The American Medical Association has adopted the position that terminating a pregnancy within the first three months should be the pregnant woman's decision. The conversations that take place between the doctor and the patient are confidential and must include offering all the necessary information from a scientific viewpoint, including the risk factors inherent in the procedure. Often, this conversation covers whether the woman has discussed it with her partner, her family, and her spiritual adviser (in the event she has one). Also, setting an appointment to see a psychotherapist before making such a difficult decision may be offered in cases in which the woman seems confused or undecided. Many gynecologists/obstetricians feel comfortable performing the procedure, especially if the mother's life is at risk; others don't. Those who do not feel comfortable because of their own religious beliefs must let the woman know this, without being judgmental about the preferences or beliefs of the patient and without imposing their own personal values.

What both the pro-choice and anti-abortion groups do agree on is that abortion should never be used as a contraceptive method. It is imperative that everyone, especially the young, be informed about how to protect themselves in order to avoid having to face this situation.

The only method to prevent pregnancy that is 100 percent foolproof is abstinence. However, there are methods with different levels of protection, including the rhythm method (which offers the least protection), condoms, diaphragms, intrauterine devices (IUDs), contraceptive pills, implants, and undergoing a vasectomy (for men) or tubal ligation (for women).

As for terminating the pregnancy, the woman makes the final decision. When performed by a qualified individual under proper conditions, the procedure involves very few risks. Statistics show that outlawing it will not lower the number of abortions; it would only increase the risk of complications, which include infections, infertility, and death in women who are subjected to the procedure or who try to perform it themselves. That is why many feel it is important that it remain a legal procedure.

THERE ARE MORE EVERY DAY

Based on calculations undertaken by the Alan Gutmacher Institute of New York, it has been estimated that, in Latin America, 4 million illegal abortions, often dangerous, are practiced annually. Even though an increasing number of women in developing countries are using contraceptives in order to have smaller families, family planning services and the ability of women to use them are inadequate and unable to achieve their goals. This study also found that the rate of abortions among Latin American women is the same or similar to that in the United States. This refutes the supposition that abortion is practiced less in predominantly Catholic countries.

For example, the report points out that, in women between the ages of fifteen and forty-nine, 2 percent of Mexican and 5 percent of Peruvian women have induced abortions every year. Also, in Brazil, there are an estimated 444 abortions per thousand pregnancies a year, with a 22.8 percent abortion rate in that country, while in Chile the percentage is 31.1 and in the Dominican Republic, 26.6. The authors of this study point out that many Latin American women "do not use contraceptives and, in fact, when they do, many become pregnant without wanting to." According to the report, women of reproductive age are in urgent need of getting better training in the use of contraceptives, especially among sexually active, single women. Dangerous abortions still play a significant role in fertility control for a vast number of Latin American women.

SINGLE MOTHERS

In the United States 21 out of every 100 babies born are the children of single mothers.

THE SINGLE MOTHER

If you are single but have decided to have a baby, even though you will be raising it without any assistance, you should know you are not alone. Even though having a child is, ideally, the product of a loving union between a couple, there are more women every day who wish to have a child outside of wedlock, either because they have not found the partner they seek or because the child's father does not want the commitment to parenthood. If this is your decision, you must feel proud of the life growing within you and ignore any prejudice from those around you.

Nor should you be concerned about how your doctor will judge you. The doctor's job is to support you and assist you during your pregnancy, regardless of your marital status. If you do not feel you are being supported, change obstetricians.

If you can, you should obtain the baby's father's family history. This will benefit your baby.

The following advice may prove helpful:

- Try to surround yourself with friends and family who appreciate and love you.
- Try not to feel alone at any time, and to know whom you can count on in case of any problem during the course of the pregnancy.
- Try to be in the company of, and sleep near, someone you trust, particularly during the final weeks, in case labor symptoms begin during the night.
- Keep your mind occupied with pleasant tasks, such as preparing the baby's clothes, readying the bedroom, and buying the proper clothing so that you continue to feel pretty, even though you've lost your waistline.

- Visit women who have young children and who have managed on their own. Their experiences will encourage and teach you.
- Do not give up activities you enjoy, as long as they do not harm the baby, such as appropriate exercising, walking on the beach or in the woods, going to the movies, or simply reading your favorite books.
- If you have not completed your studies, try to continue them as long as your condition allows. More than ever, you will need to be professionally prepared so that you can meet your needs and those of your baby.
- And do not forget, your baby needs a happy mother, one who is capable of taking on the responsibilities his or her father has run away from. After all, it's better to be alone than in bad company!

WORLD'S PREEMIEST PREEMIE

The world's most premature baby was James Elgin Gill, born in Ottawa, Canada, on May 20, 1987, 128 days after conception, weighing one pound, six ounces.

MULTIPLE PREGNANCIES

Pregnancies including twins, triplets, or more babies have increased significantly. This is partly due to several medications used in infertility cases, such as Clomid or Pergonal, as well as to in vitro (or test-tube) fertilization techniques. Although twins may be detected during the second trimester due to the rapid growth and size of the abdomen, an ultrasound will confirm the presence of two (or more) infants because it shows their images.

A very large womb at a certain stage of pregnancy may represent not a multiple pregnancy, but an excess of amniotic fluid, fibromas (benign tumors in the womb), an enlarged ovary, etc. Thanks to ultrasound, mothers today need not wait—as my sister did with her first pregnancy—to find out if it was one very large child or twins. When she was in her eighth month, and ultrasound was still not available, she did not know if it would be a large baby (as was the case with her son) or twins.

Multiple pregnancies slightly increase the risk of complications for the baby as well as for the mother. As for the infants, there is a higher risk of miscarriage or death, deformities, growth retardation, and low birth weight. As for the mother, the complications can include, among others, the following: anemia, preeclampsia, tearing of the placenta, placenta previa, hemorrhages, premature delivery, complicated delivery due to the position of the infants at the moment of delivery, and twisting of the infants' umbilical cords.

The most common problem in multiple pregnancies is premature delivery. The more babies that are in the mother's womb, the shorter the gestation period and the less the babies weigh at birth. Calculations for a single pregnancy period are between thirty-seven and forty weeks; for a double pregnancy about thirty-six to thirty-seven, for triplets only thirty-five. This means that the babies have less opportunity to grow, develop, and mature within the uterus. This could cause complications, which might even require temporary admission to an intensive care facility. That is why doctors insist on bringing every pregnancy to term, as long as neither the mother nor the baby is in danger. Often, absolute rest is recommended in the final months of the pregnancy.

Heredity is another factor in the event of multiple pregnancies, at least with twins. Some suggest that women who have a twin brother or sister have a greater chance of having twins, as do their granddaughters. The incidence is one in every ninety births in the United States. The cases of triplets are less frequent, occurring once in every 9,000 births.

Ideally, all pregnant women, but especially those expecting more than one baby, must follow a healthy and balanced diet and should consider adjusting their intake of calories, since they will be required to feed more than one baby. Your doctor can advise you or refer you to a dietitian. The same is true of vitamins and minerals. Your doctor may also recommend some medication to relax the uterus (Ritodrine, for instance) if there is any danger of a premature delivery.

CRISTINA SARALEGUI
Hostess of *El show de Cristina* and journalist

When my son Jon Marcos was born—eleven years ago—I was already thirty-nine. Because of my age, I had an amniocentesis and an ultrasound. When I was having my ultrasound, I realized that the nurses and the technicians had noticed something unusual, but they wouldn't tell me or my husband, Marcos, anything. There was a big to-do in the ultrasound room!

The physician told me that I had "something" on the ultrasound, but that he couldn't tell me anything else because he wasn't sure of what it was, and that any surgical procedure could damage the baby. The end result was that I had to wait the nine months of pregnancy with that "something" inside of me. Finally, when I delivered, we found out that what I had was a fibromyoma. In spite of the fact that it was benign, it had grown significantly. I think that Jon Marcos was born three weeks early because he was tired of sharing his space with it!

What I learned from my first pregnancy that was helpful for the second one is that it's important to control what you eat. If you don't control your diet when you are pregnant, you become a house on wheels and the baby can become too heavy. My first child, Cristina Amalia (we call her Titi), who is currently nineteen years old, weighed more than ten pounds at birth. That's why I made a promise to myself that with the second pregnancy I would not gain as much weight. Babies need to put on weight outside the tummy, not inside.

A big mistake with my second pregnancy was that, after gaining fifty pounds, I put myself on a very fast and strict diet after delivery. I wanted Marcos, my husband, to see that I was back in shape immediately. And thanks to the diet, I did lose the fifty pounds in four months, but it affected my health with problems that continued for a long time. I do not recommend that any new mother put herself on these kinds of drastic diets!

With both of my pregnancies I worked until the day I delivered. I remember that when I was in my last month with Jon Marcos, my husband picked me up at work to eat lunch. After eating, I got so sleepy that I couldn't return to work and had to go home to rest for a while to see if my drowsiness would go away. I lay down to take a nap, and when I woke up, I was giving birth!

During the last few months of pregnancy, I had to travel a lot, and each time I was on a plane I got motion sickness and had to go to the bathroom to throw up. But my tummy was so big that I had to vomit with the door open, because the airplane's bathroom was too small. And everybody saw me: very professional, dressed as an executive, and throwing up with the door open.

My recommendation for your first pregnancy is not to listen to your friends' or relatives' advice. Listen only to your doctor. Friends fill our heads with stories that if it hurts, you should take this or do that. Don't pay attention to any of that; it's better to follow your physician's recommendations and read professionally written books on pregnancy.

Chapter 2

YOUR HEALTH

Even though each pregnancy is unique, in general terms, your first pregnancy is an example of how the next ones will take place. There is, however, always the possibility that a second pregnancy will be less complicated than the first. We should also take into consideration that a woman is more prepared to confront a second pregnancy, since she already has an idea of the situations she will experience and how to deal with them.

Some of the most frequently asked questions by my patients or women writing to me are related to their concerns about what will happen during pregnancy and how they must care for themselves.

One of the things that helps the most in ensuring a comfortable and uncomplicated pregnancy is a future mother who is in good overall health. As I have mentioned earlier, if you suffer from any acute or chronic health problem, placing yourself under constant medical supervision during the pregnancy is extremely important. Under ideal circumstances, eliminate problems that can be eliminated (for example, taking care of an infection such as vaginitis) and control those that need to be controlled (such as sugar levels in your blood, in the case of diabetes), even before conception. Other recommendations that may help increase the enjoyment of those nine months include the following tips.

TIPS TO HELP YOU ENJOY YOUR PREGNANCY

- Watch your diet. Proper nutrition will help the baby's development and keep you in good shape (see Chapter 4 on diet and exercise).
- Try to reduce the stress in your life. Mental health is as important as physical health. This is the moment to find someone who will help with your chores at home or with your other children, and who will afford you the chance to get the rest your body needs in this phase of your life.
- Avoid gaining more than twenty-five pounds (twelve kilos) during the nine-month period, and try to gain them gradually. This way you will avoid having to diet toward the end because you gained too much during the first months.
- Exercise regularly (see Chapter 4 for exercise recommendations).

YOUR MEDICAL AND GYNECOLOGICAL HISTORY

Information on your medical history is as important to your obstetrician as the information he or she obtains at each visit throughout the development of the pregnancy (see Chapter 1).

PREVIOUS ABORTIONS

Previous abortions may have been spontaneous (miscarriages) or induced. A prior history of miscarriage may prompt the doctor to request certain tests and take certain precautions.

In general, a history of induced abortion, especially during the first three months, presents no particular risk. Especially if it was performed after 1973, when the procedure was legalized in the United States. If an abortion was performed when the pregnancy was more advanced (after the first three months), there is a small chance that the neck of the womb could have weakened, which the doctor will monitor carefully.

In the event a woman has an Rh-negative blood type, if there was a pregnancy and/or previous abortion (miscarriage or induced), it is important to check for antibodies against the Rh factor that may have been formed when exposed to the red blood cells of the previous fetus. Based on this, your doctor will give you an injection or take other precautions to protect your baby from developing related problems. (For further details, see "blood incompatibility" later in this chapter.)

> **"I am afraid I may have a miscarriage because I am thirty-eight years old and my only previous pregnancy ended in a miscarriage. Should I remain in bed during the first three months?"**

Although it is true that when you have had a previous pregnancy or when you are over thirty-five the risk of a miscarriage increases, most women carry their pregnancies to term. Women between thirty and forty years of age have a higher propensity to miscarriage than those between twenty and thirty, but less than women over forty. This is due to a higher incidence of abnormalities in the chromosomes (one of the components in the ova) of women over thirty-five. These abnormalities may cause fetal defects that are incompatible with life, so nature does not allow them to develop. There are other causes for spontaneous abortions, such as hormonal problems, and your doctor will most certainly take blood tests to evaluate them (for example, thyroid tests). Occasionally, progesterone may be prescribed.

Not all cases require complete rest. Depending on your particular case, your doctor could recommend decreasing your physical activities, resting more, and avoiding sexual intercourse during the first three months. The risk of a miscarriage decreases after eight weeks of pregnancy and is even lower once the first trimester has been completed.

Many times I remind my patients that there are women who have attempted to interrupt pregnancy by extreme exercising—running, riding—or have had car accidents or fallen off a horse without achieving the loss of the fetus or the abortion.

PROBABILITY OF CONCEIVING

Even under optimum conditions, the probability of a couple conceiving on any given month throughout the year is one in five.

FIBROIDS

Fibroids or uterine fibromyomas are benign tumors of the womb. They are found mostly in women over thirty-five and are more common today since an increasing number of women in that age range are becoming pregnant. In most cases, their presence causes no problems. However, they have occasionally been linked to infertility.

There are different types of fibroid tumors. They may vary in size from very small to very large. They can be found outside the womb (known as subserous), in the muscle tissue of the womb (known as intramural), or within the uterine cavity (known as submucous). Intramural and submucous fibromyomas are the most dangerous during pregnancy. They usually cause no symptoms and are diagnosed during the physical examination or the ultrasound test.

Although most women who have fibroids do not have problems during their deliveries, occasionally their presence can slightly increase the risk of an ectopic pregnancy, a low placenta, the premature separation of the placenta from the wall of the uterus (the womb), a premature delivery, or other complications as described later.

If you are aware you have them, report it to your doctor. If you are unaware, your doctor may discover them during the initial examination or later on. Other complications caused by fibroids include abdominal pain or pressure on other organs. Occasionally, if a woman has had previous surgery to remove fibroid tumors, or depending on their location or size, the doctor may suggest, depending on your specific case, a cesarean section instead of vaginal delivery.

> "Is it possible the fibroids may grow and make me lose my baby? They appeared after my second delivery. Do you recommend that I have them removed before I become pregnant again?"

Not all women with fibroids are at a higher risk of losing their baby. Many factors are involved. Yes, they can be removed before a pregnancy, but this is not always necessary. Depending on their size, fibroids may alter the shape of the womb. Since they are made of a fibrous tissue, they lack the number of blood vessels normally present in the healthy womb tissue. If the fertilized ova nestles in the area of the fibromyoma or if the placenta grows in this area, it is possible the fetus will not receive enough blood to grow and could therefore be lost. Fibroid tumors tend to increase in size during pregnancy due to the high level of female hormones. If this causes the uterus to grow abnormally, it may cause an abortion in the second trimester or a premature delivery. You must notify your doctor in the event of bleeding or premature contractions, since there is medication available to arrest premature labor.

Concerning the issue of removing the fibroids before pregnancy, it is important to determine their exact size and location. Intramural and submucous fibromyomas are the ones that may cause problems more frequently. There are several procedures in which only the fibroid is removed, such as myomectomy, uterine artery embolization, and MRI-guided focused ultrasound surgery. If a hysterectomy is recommended (complete removal of the womb) due to fibroids, make sure you get a second opinion before undergoing the procedure. I have had various patients who have managed to carry pregnancies to term without complications in spite of the presence of fibroids and others who have done so following a myomectomy.

INCOMPETENT CERVIX

The neck of the uterus, known as the cervix, may be weakened due to a previous abortion during the second trimester of pregnancy or simply due to genetic reasons (hereditary or congenital). This condition is known as "incompetent" cervix. Its presence can cause an abortion during the second trimester of pregnancy. Unfortunately, that is often the way in which it is diagnosed. The woman may suddenly develop dilation of the cervix without any pain, contractions, bleeding, or any other symptoms, and may lose the baby. When there is a prior history of this problem, or it is suspected for some reason, the doctor may stitch (suture) the cervix, to make it narrower, at the beginning of the second trimester. These sutures are eliminated a few weeks before delivery or when labor starts.

Occasionally in these cases, the doctor will forbid sexual intercourse during the duration of the pregnancy and sometimes will recommend complete rest or the use of a special instrument that bolsters the uterus.

MASSAGING IS FINE, BUT BEWARE OF *HUESEROS* (UNLICENSED CHIROPRACTORS)

Hueseros are people who, without a formal education, like *curanderos* (healers), treat certain "ailments" related to aching bones and muscles. They are a sort of unlicensed chiropractor. I have patients who swear they have been helped by them. My advice, during pregnancy, is that conventional massaging (not too deep) without cracking of the bones presents no problem. But avoid contortions, rough manipulations, or bone cracking.

PREVIOUS PREGNANCIES

Frequently, a woman who has had a difficult first delivery manages the second one with a lot more ease, especially if the complications of the first were due to specific causes such as an infection or an uncontrolled disease like diabetes, which may be prevented or more adequately treated the second time around. Although there are no guarantees, to increase the possibility of easy delivery it is absolutely necessary to talk with your obstetrician to define the strategy you will follow and the goals you wish to reach.

Obviously, circumstances exist that cannot be predicted and/or prevented, such as a baby's position at the moment of delivery that does not allow a vaginal birth. However, the general consensus is that the second and subsequent pregnancies benefit from the advantage of encountering a more relaxed birthing canal, a more experienced mother, and a shorter period of labor.

In the case of women who have had previous cesareans, notifying their doctor and arriving early at the hospital when they notice the beginning of labor symptoms is important. The scar, or scars, of previous cesareans may slightly increase the risk of a ruptured womb during contractions, and the situation requires constant medical supervision.

This does not mean that all women who have already undergone a cesarean section will necessarily require one in subsequent pregnancies, which was the thinking until recently. Actually, many women have managed vaginal deliveries without any problems after having previously undergone a cesarean section. Your doctor will advise you in your particular case what is most beneficial to you and your baby. Frequently, that decision is made during labor.

MYTH: IF THE BABY MOVES A LOT, IT IS A BOY; IF IT IS CALMER, IT IS A GIRL

This reminds me of mothers who say that boys are always more active than girls. I remember that when my nephew was born, my sister and I could talk on the telephone uninterrupted for quite a while because he would be entertained by any toy and would remain quietly seated. On the other hand, as soon as my little niece started crawling, it was impossible to leave her alone for even two minutes, because she immediately would be climbing on a chair or a table. On one occasion, while I was talking with my sister, she was trying to climb into the oven which, happily, had been turned off.

The same applies to movements within the uterus. The fact that the unborn child is more active does not mean that it's a soccer player or a boy. Moreover, the perception of movement varies from one woman to another. Women who have already had a child tend to be more sensitive to subsequent babies' movements. This is also true in slimmer women. Lastly, the detection of movement also depends on the baby's position within the womb.

IN VITRO FERTILIZATION

Every day more women are undergoing test-tube or in vitro fertilization, for different reasons. The most common of these relate to infertility problems. Generally, the risks during the pregnancy are similar to those in a pregnancy stemming from natural sexual intercourse. Occasionally, the doctor may suggest certain extra precautions in the initial stages, such as temporarily abstaining from sexual relations and vigorous exercising, and may suggest taking progesterone (a hormone that increases the possibilities of the egg implanting and remaing adhered to the placenta). As in the case in which medication is used to induce ovulation, a slight increase in the incidence of these women producing twins or triplets is noted (between five and twenty-five of every one hundred pregnancies obtained through in vitro fertilization). In this event, the woman must take the same precautions as a woman with a multiple pregnancy (see Chapter 1, multiple pregnancies).

INCIDENCE OF PREGNANCY

- Between 60 and 80 percent of the women who do not use any birth-control methods will become pregnant in the course of a year after having engaged in regular sexual intercourse.
- Almost 14 percent of North American couples using condoms find that, despite their precautions, involuntary pregnancies occur, something that is frequently due to incorrect use of the condom.
- Of women who trust the man to remove his penis before ejaculating and who think they will avoid becoming pregnant, 25 percent do become pregnant.

PAST MEDICAL HISTORY
OF THE FATHER AND BOTH FAMILIES

During the last few years we have learned that the age and health of the father may also have an important effect on the baby's future. For example, it has been found that there is a greater incidence of Down's syndrome in babies whose fathers are over fifty. Intrauterine growth may also be delayed in babies whose fathers abuse alcohol. Just to think that, for centuries, men have blamed women for all problems related to pregnancy and delivery!

It's also important to realize that many families, especially Hispanic ones, hide abortions, whether spontaneous or induced, or the death of babies during delivery or within a few days of birth. Your knowledge of family history concerning miscarriages, premature births, or stillborn babies is very important.

The couple must be informed about the existence of genetic defects in both families. Sometimes families prefer not to mention them, because they are ashamed, but this information is absolutely necessary to determine whether certain tests are required, and to prevent or control hereditary problems. In order to obtain this information, talk openly and honestly with your close relatives.

BEWARE OF HERBS AND TEAS!

Although part of our Hispanic tradition involves asking your neighbor or *comadre* (close friend) about the use of herbs and teas for almost any ailment, when you are pregnant or breast-feeding, you must be extremely cautious. Did you know that some herbs that are sold in the United States come into the country as veterinary preparations so that Customs doesn't check them? Did you know that sometimes these herbs are contaminated with animal feces because their preparation does not always follow proper sanitary regulations? Did you know that there are herbs and teas that can cause an abortion? Did you know that some of these products can reach your baby through your milk and harm it? There are some wonderful preparations, but before you take any herbs or teas, check with your doctor. And, if there is any question, do not take them during pregnancy or while breast-feeding.

BLOOD INCOMPATIBILITY (RH FACTOR)

One of the first tests you will undergo during pregnancy is a blood test to determine the presence of the mother's Rh factor. Normally we have a blood type that can be O, A, B, etc., and that is either Rh positive or Rh negative. Most people have the Rh factor (in other words, it is positive). Approximately 15 percent of women and 15 percent of men do not have it (it is negative). If both parents are Rh positive or both are Rh negative, there are no incompatibility issues with the baby's blood.

But, if the mother is Rh negative and the baby is Rh positive, the mother may develop antibodies against the baby's Rh factor during the delivery. This is because a certain amount of the baby's blood goes into the mother's bloodstream, which is not accustomed to the "invading" Rh factor. This causes the woman to produce antibodies (as if she were fighting an intruder in her body). If she were to become pregnant again and the second baby were also Rh positive, these antibodies might attempt to destroy the baby's red blood cells. This is called blood incompatibility. In severe cases, the baby may require blood transfusions during pregnancy (within the womb) or at birth.

Today, thanks to scientific advancements, this can be prevented. A substance, known as human anti-Rh gamma globulin (Rhogam), prevents antibodies from being formed and prevents blood incompatibility problems. It is generally recommended during the twenty-eighth week of gestation and during the first seventy-two hours after delivery. This injection is also recommended in cases of previous miscarriages or abortions, or when the mother is Rh negative (unless the father is known to be Rh negative).

BABIES . . . AFTER FORTY

Many women, once they reach forty, think they no longer need to worry about becoming pregnant. But this is not the case, since women close to menopause also have unwanted pregnancies, although less frequently than younger women. According to Dr. Kirtly Parker Jones of the School of Medicine at the University of Utah, older women should know that they have the same birth-control alternatives as younger women and they should use them.

A PREGNANCY AFTER THIRTY-FIVE

Until a few years ago, cases of women over thirty-five becoming pregnant for the first time were the exception to the rule. Today, however, this is becoming increasingly common. Many women prefer to study and have a career and be prepared for their futures before facing maternity. Although advances in obstetrics have reduced the risk of problems in pregnancies for these women, there is still a slight increase in the risk of complications within this age-group. As with all other aspects of life, there are advantages and disadvantages to delaying motherhood.

RISKS (DOWN'S SYNDROME, HYPERTENSION, DIABETES, ETC.)

The disadvantages of delaying conception include a decrease in fertility with age. Some women experience more problems getting pregnant after they are thirty-five. And, although science and its progress offer a lot of help in this regard, the risk of some congenital deformities increases with age—specifically Down's syndrome, which we mentioned in the case of fathers over fifty. The risk of an older woman having a Down's baby is much higher than that of an older man.

DOWN'S SYNDROME

Statistics show that the risk of having a child with Down's syndrome increases proportionately with age: at twenty, only 1 of 10,000 pregnant women run this risk, at thirty-five the risk increases to 3 out of every 1,000. At forty, the risk factor is 1 out of every 100.

Although the difficult decision to continue or terminate a pregnancy when it is known that the baby is a Down's syndrome child is up to the parents, doctors routinely recommend that all women thirty-five and over, as well as women who have other risk factors (previous problems or family history), undergo prenatal diagnostic testing to find out whether the infant carries this or other problems. According to some studies, only 10 percent of children born with Down's syndrome have serious mental retardation and other medical problems. Many enjoy long and happy lives.

Another risk for mothers over thirty-five—especially those who are overweight—is the higher probability of developing high blood pressure, heart disease, diabetes, premature delivery miscarriage, and postpartum hemorrhage.

Modern technology—using early testing, such as amniocentesis and a sample of chorionic tissue (described in Chapter 3)—may detect a large number of fetal defects within the first three months. The ultrasound monitoring during pregnancy, electronic monitoring of the baby during labor, close supervision of the woman to control diabetes, blood pressure, and other medical problems, as well as early induction of labor when considered necessary, have been able to considerably reduce problems in high-risk women (which includes women over thirty-five).

Obviously, the woman's participation is essential in order to reduce risk factors. I am referring to her awareness regarding her diet, exercise, and prenatal supervision.

AND YOU THINK YOU HAVE A LARGE FAMILY!

- The world's record for births is held by a Russian peasant woman, the wife of Feodor Vassiliev, who gave birth to sixty-nine children, all multiple births, including sixteen pairs of twins, seven sets of triplets, and four sets of quadruplets. The case was reported in 1782. Only two of Mrs. Vassiliev's children died in infancy.
- In Latin America, the record is held by Leontina Albina Espinosa, of San Antonio, Chile, who gave birth to her fifty-fifth son (her last) in 1981. Only forty children survived.

THE ADVANTAGE OF AGE

Many people think that the loudly proclaimed—and, to some extent, exaggerated—risks of mothers thirty-five and over are compensated for by the advantages a baby born to a mature, balanced, and experienced mother has, compared to a baby born of a teenager or of someone in her twenties who is in the midst of developing a career. Studies have shown that older mothers tend to be more patient with their children, to know more about educating them and—in spite of the fact that their physical energy may not equal that of a younger woman—to never regret becoming mothers.

An extremely popular myth is that, when a woman turns thirty-five, her possibilities of having a child with Down's syndrome increase considerably. In fact, those risks begin increasing after twenty . . . but not very significantly until after forty, as I have already pointed out.

In any case, most doctors—since it is better to be safe than sorry—advise their pregnant patients who are between thirty-five and forty, or who are close to being thirty-five, to undergo prenatal testing to ensure that the baby is healthy.

A WOMAN'S LIFESTYLE CHOICES
THAT MAY COMPLICATE PREGNANCY

- Smoking
- Drinking alcoholic beverages
- Using drugs
- Taking nonprescribed medications
- Being malnourished (having bad nutrition habits or not gaining sufficient weight during the pregnancy)
- Using certain herbs or teas without prior medical consultation (such as *ma huang* and others)
- Not getting prenatal care

MEDICAL PROBLEMS THAT MAY COMPLICATE A PREGNANCY

- Infections
- Diabetes
- Hypertension
- Kidney, liver, lung, or heart disease
- Severe anemia

OBSTETRICAL SITUATIONS THAT MAY COMPLICATE A PREGNANCY

- Pregnancy in women under fifteen years of age
- Pregnancy in women over thirty-five years of age
- Complications with previous pregnancies
- Development of gestational diabetes
- Children with congenital diseases (at birth)
- Multiple pregnancies (twins, triplets, etc.)
- Delay in the normal growth of the baby in the womb
- Premature babies
- Bleeding, especially during the second or third trimester of the pregnancy
- Eclampsia or preeclampsia (high blood pressure in the mother as she reaches term)
- Abnormal heartbeat in the baby

MARÍA ELENA SALINAS
Univisión newscaster

My daughter is named Julia Alexandra Rodríguez. She was born on the first of November, 1994. I didn't experience much discomfort during my first pregnancy. The worst thing was that, during the last few months, I swelled up a lot due to the fact that I was retaining so much liquid, something I attribute to my bad habit of eating too much salt.

Since I had already had two miscarriages before having Julia, just the fact of being able to get pregnant again was a wonderful experience. Perhaps the best thing that happened to me during the pregnancy was that it gave me a great sense of inner peace. Having a baby inside me helped to put my life in perspective and made me realize that the things I worried about before weren't really that important.

The most impressive moment of all for me was seeing my baby during the ultrasound tests. It was so hard to believe that a little being was growing inside of me! When she was born, I couldn't believe how much she resembled the image in the ultrasound.

I learned something during my first pregnancy that helped me a lot during my second:* the importance of staying on a diet to prevent me from gaining too much weight and of doing a little exercise so I wouldn't feel so bloated. I also found it useful to read all the books on pregnancy that I could, because they helped me to know what was going on inside me, and what to expect.

My first daughter was delivered by C-section, since the baby was in breech position and my doctor thought it was too dangerous to try to turn her around. But I had a very bad experience with the cesarean as the incision got infected and I had to stay in bed for a month following the delivery. I would've preferred twenty-four hours of pain to a month of suffering! If it's possible, I'd like to have my second child by natural birth.

*At the time of this interview, María Elena Salinas was in the third trimester of her second pregnancy.

Based on my own experience, I'd like to tell women who are going through their first pregnancy to take good care of themselves and not to pay attention to people who say, "My mother drank, smoked, and ate what she wanted during her pregnancy and had me with no problems at all." They were lucky things turned out well! Now that we are more informed about the risks of pregnancy, what does it matter if you sacrifice your lifestyle for nine or ten months in order to ensure that your baby will be healthy and that you will have a problem-free delivery?

I would also suggest that women who are pregnant for the first time try to be patient, even if they find it difficult. It is not easy enduring sleepless nights, listening to crying that goes on forever, and understanding how defenseless and how dependent on us, their parents, these tiny newborns are.

Chapter 3

RISKS TO PREGNANCY

SEXUALLY TRANSMITTED DISEASES

These diseases are also known as venereal diseases, and they can occur at any time, not only during pregnancy. Unfortunately, their incidence has increased during the last ten years. The consequences could be greater if contracted during pregnancy because they could affect not only the health of the pregnant woman, but of her baby as well.

Pregnant or not, when you have only one sexual partner and that partner has an exclusive relationship with you, the risks of transmitting these diseases obviously decrease dramatically. Nevertheless, some venereal diseases might have been contracted before the monogamous relationship began and can manifest months, or even years, later. These include the viral infection known as HIV (AIDS) and genital herpes. On many occasions, these and other infections may be asymptomatic.

Women who have more than one partner or think that their partner might be having intimate sexual contact with other people (men or women) can protect themselves from these diseases (to a great degree) through the use of a condom. Knowledge of signs and symptoms is important because they might alert you to a problem. If you don't have symptoms but think you might have been exposed anyway, it's important to tell your doctor so he or she can perform the necessary tests and treat the disease.

GONORRHEA

Gonorrhea is highly contagious. Frequently (although not always), the male notices a yellowish discharge and experiences difficulty urinating. The signs of infection in the woman may be absent or manifest themselves as a yellowish vaginal discharge and, sometimes, as pain in the lower abdomen. If this occurs during the pregnancy and remains untreated, it could cause conjunctivitis, blindness, and a generalized infection in the fetus.

GENITAL HERPES

Genital herpes can be transmitted to the baby upon delivery, when it passes through the birth canal, if there is an active outbreak of the infection at the time of birth. Although the risk of infection isn't very high, it could be very serious for the baby if he or she were to contract the infection.

HERPES: THE GOOD AND THE BAD

It's possible for a man or a woman to have sexual intercourse several times with a person who is infected with the genital herpes virus, yet never contract it. But a woman who is not infected could contract the virus of an infected partner at the least convenient time in her life: when she is pregnant. If the genital herpes virus is transmitted to the baby during birth, it could cause serious diseases in the child and even death. Therefore, if a woman has an outbreak of herpes when she is about to give birth, a cesarean section will performed. In that way, the baby will not be infected.

SYPHILIS

A woman who contracts syphilis can pass the infection on to the baby if she goes untreated. The consequences for the baby could be serious, including, among others: bone deformities, damage to the nervous system, and even stillbirths. These dangers can be avoided by taking antibiotics in the early stages of pregnancy.

CHLAMYDIA

This is the most frequent venereal disease in the United States. If the pregnant woman has had several sexual partners, her doctor might recommend that he or she take a culture (a test of the urethral or vaginal fluid that looks specifically for chlamydia) in order to rule out that infection. Often this disease does not cause any symptoms. If chlamydia goes untreated, the baby might develop a pulmonary infection or an infection in the eyes.

MYTH: YOU HAVE TO EAT FOR TWO

There is some truth to this, since now you have a little baby inside . . . but the baby is very small and only needs the equivalent of 300 to 500 extra calories a day. In addition, at this stage, the baby needs food that give it the calcium, iron, proteins, and vitamins that will enable it to grow in a healthy way. It doesn't need sweet rolls with chocolate, or *churros*, or fried foods. The pregnant woman should ideally gain a maximum of twenty-five pounds (or twelve kilos) during the nine months . . . after all, she is giving birth to a baby, not an adult.

VAGINITIS

Vaginitis means "vaginal inflammation," and it is not always due to sexual contact with an infected partner. In addition, it doesn't necessarily cause any symptoms. Its causes are varied. When it is due to an infection, it should be treated with antibiotics. The more common infections are caused by certain bacterias known as *Gardnerella* (also called *Hemophilus*) and *Streptococcus*. Detecting them is very simple, but your doctor should examine a sample of vaginal fluid under a microscope or send it to the laboratory. Treatment is important in order to prevent spreading the infection to the baby (like pneumonia) and/or premature rupture of the membranes that surround the baby, among other complications.

GENITAL WARTS

Genital warts are growths (generally benign) caused by a virus known as human papillomavirus infection, abbreviated HPV. When they are very large, they can block or narrow the birth canal, requiring a cesarean delivery. They can occasionally be transmitted to the baby.

HIV/AIDS

The chances of having contracted the HIV virus, or AIDS, increase if you have had several sexual partners, if you or your partner have used intravenous drugs, if your sexual partner has had sexual intercourse with another man, or if you have had blood transfusions (especially prior to 1984, when they began to do HIV testing on blood). In cases in which the woman is infected with HIV, she can transmit it to the baby either during pregnancy or at the time of birth. Although we do not have a way of eliminating the virus from the body at this time, there are various studies that show that if the mother is diagnosed early on, certain treatments can significantly decrease the risk of transmitting the virus to the baby. If there is a possibility that you have been exposed to HIV, take the test, preferably before getting pregnant.

"I am three months pregnant and I feel fine. Although I know my husband loves me very much, I'm worried that he may not always be faithful to me. Could this pose a risk to the baby? Is there something I can do to protect the baby?"

Ideally, you should be able to talk to your husband, have him reassure you that he is only with you, and believe him. If that isn't the case, in order to protect your baby you could use latex condoms when you have sexual intercourse. Even though they don't provide a 100 percent guarantee, they offer you more protection than using nothing at all. If you didn't have an HIV test before becoming pregnant, or during the pregnancy, ask your doctor to do one (for your peace of mind). Even though there might be a period of up to six months between possible exposure to the virus and the blood test coming back positive, if it shows negative, it would be less likely that you've been infected. It can always be repeated in a few months. Share your concern with your obstetrician as well, who will do additional tests if he or she considers it necessary.

HEPATITIS B AND C

Hepatitis B and C are infections caused by two different types of virus. They can be transmitted by sexual intercourse or by exposure to infected blood. In the United States, blood banks regularly test for both to prevent transmission through blood transfusions. These diseases can damage the mother's liver. If contracted during pregnancy—especially hepatitis B—they could cause damage to the baby's liver too. In severe cases, they may even cause the baby's death. Hepatitis B infection is more than 95 percent preventable if exposed babies receive hepatitis B immunoglobulin and hepatitis B vaccine at birth. Your doctor will test you for hepatitis B surface antigen (a blood test) to detect infection and ensure proper prophylaxis of your baby if necessary. The risk of hepatitis C transmission to the baby during pregnancy seems to be small, except in women who are also infected with the HIV virus. At this time we do not have an effective hepatitis C vaccine or immunoglobulin.

GENETIC DEFECTS

Skin color, hair texture, eye color, facial features, height, etc., are some of the characteristics we receive from our parents, at the time of conception, through our genes. The combination of the father's and mother's genes constitute the baby's genetic inheritance, which, in time, will also be transmitted to his or her children.

Unfortunately, along with the good, we can also inherit the bad. Sometimes it takes only one defective gene to develop into a disease in the baby. That is why marriages between close relatives have four times the risk of hereditary diseases compared to marriages between unrelated couples.

GENETIC PREDISPOSITION

When one of the parents has a dominant gene for a certain disease, there is a 50 percent risk that each one of his children will manifest that defect.

There are some tests that can be done to detect certain genetic problems in the baby. If your doctor feels that this is warranted in your case, he or she will suggest that you have one or more tests for prenatal detection. In certain instances your doctor will refer you to a geneticist, who will explain what the risks are in having a child with a certain hereditary or genetic defect and how much information can be obtained through different tests. Risks are increased in the following cases:

- Women over thirty-five and men over fifty. As I mentioned before, they run a higher risk of having a child with Down's syndrome.
- Couples who have had a child with a genetic defect or families whose close relatives have had children with genetic defects.
- Women with a history of repeated miscarriages or of stillbirths.
- Couples who belong to certain groups that have a greater predisposition toward carrying genes for certain diseases. For example, Tay-Sachs disease, which predominantly affects people of Jewish descent from Central and Eastern Europe; or sickle cell anemia, in African-American patients.

ECTOPIC PREGNANCY

An ectopic pregnancy means that the fetus is not growing in the uterus but in another part of the woman's body, almost always in one of the fallopian tubes. The risk in these cases is that these tubes are not made to expand with the growth of the fetus and, if the pregnancy is not detected early on, can rupture, causing internal abdominal bleeding. Fortunately, the majority of ectopic pregnancies are diagnosed before they can cause problems. Their symptoms are very characteristic: a sharp and sudden abdominal pain and/or vaginal bleeding. It is a medical emergency. It is treated surgically by removing the embryo from the tube. Sometimes it's necessary to remove the tube as well.

WHICH WOMEN RUN A GREATER RISK OF HAVING AN ECTOPIC PREGNANCY?

- Women who have had pelvic infections
- Women who suffer from endometriosis
- Women who become pregnant in spite of having an intrauterine device (IUD)
- Women who have had their fallopian tubes operated on

OTHER RISKS

MISCARRIAGE

The great majority of miscarriages, or noninduced abortions, take place before the pregnancy reaches the sixteenth week, especially around the eighth week. More than half of the pregnancies that do not come to term are the result of problems with the embryo or fetus that prevent normal development (for example, malformations of the chromosomes, which are part of the genes, found in the ovum and the spermatozoa that form the egg). The rest are due to maternal complications or circumstances in which the cause is unknown.

When the fetus develops normally, there are maternal factors that still might cause or contribute to a miscarriage. Among them are

- Chronic diseases in the mother
- Malformation of the uterus
- Uterine fibroid tumors
- Low progesterone (a hormone in the blood)
- Stress
- High fever for a prolonged period of time
- Bruises, lesions, or accidents in general
- A weakness in the cervix, which causes it to open before the pregnancy has come to term; this happens especially in the second trimester

When faced with the threat of miscarriage, above all, remain calm. Many symptoms that might be those of miscarriage are nothing more than the normal discomfort of pregnancy. Nevertheless, if you notice any of the following symptoms, you should call your doctor immediately:

- If you have bleeding along with cramps in the lower part of the abdomen
- If you have severe pain, even though you are not bleeding
- If you are bleeding a lot, as though you were menstruating, or if you are spotting for several consecutive days
- If the bleeding is heavy enough that you have to change sanitary pads every hour; this is an emergency, and you should call for help

POSSIBILITY OF MISCARRIAGE

The possibility of miscarriage increases with the age of the pregnant woman. While the risk is around 12 to 15 percent for a woman around age twenty, a forty-year-old woman's risk is 25 percent.

ANEMIA

This is a deficiency in the number of red blood cells (which could cause increased fatigue). Even though this may have several causes, the most common is iron deficiency. This is why it is recommended that women eat food containing iron and take prenatal vitamins.

IRON PRESCRIPTION MEDICINES, SUPPLEMENTS

Although they are sold without prescription, do not take any supplement or product, whether herbal, vitamin, mineral, etc., without consulting your doctor. This includes melatonin, ginger, diet teas, laxatives, etc. For example, ginger is recommended by some obstetricians to control nausea during the first three months of pregnancy, but others recommend a certain maximum dose per day. For this reason, during the pregnancy and while breast-feeding—even though they may have worked for a friend and she recommends them—don't take these products without consulting your doctor.

DIABETES AND GESTATIONAL DIABETES

Diabetes refers to an elevation of the blood sugar or blood glucose above normal levels. There is a difference between a woman who is a known diabetic and decides to become pregnant and a woman who develops diabetes during pregnancy; this is known as gestational diabetes. Gestational diabetes is a temporary condition that clears up once the pregnancy is over. About 2 to 5 percent of women develop gestational diabetes in the

United States. It usually develops in the last half of the pregnancy when the hormones made by the placenta counteract the effect of insulin, a hormone produced by the pancreas (an organ in the abdomen).

WHO IS MOST LIKELY TO GET DIABETES?

- People who are overweight
- People with a family history of diabetes
- People who are forty and older
- Hispanics, Native Americans, and African Americans
- Women who have delivered a baby of 9 pounds or more

Even though a woman with gestational diabetes has a higher risk of developing diabetes in the future, her blood sugars are easier to control during pregnancy and go back to normal after delivery. In the case of either form of diabetes, it is of extreme importance to try to control the levels of blood sugar to prevent complications.

The diagnosis is established with fasting blood sugars. A screening test at twenty-four to twenty-eight weeks of pregnancy is recommended. This is done by giving the pregnant woman fifty grams of sugar in a drink and taking a blood sample one or two hours later. When in doubt, a glucose tolerance test follows. Early detection and appropriate management will avoid potential problems for mother and baby.

The treatment may consist of diet and exercise. Sometimes insulin is needed as well. During pregnancy oral hypoglycemics (diabetes pills) are not recommended. This means that if a woman was taking them before getting pregnant, she will need to switch to insulin during the pregnancy.

Complications during delivery, and in the first days of the baby's life, include a more difficult labor if the baby is very large (especially if the mother is petite) or a need to do a cesarean. The baby may experience hypoglycemia (low blood sugar) during the first few days or may be premature.

BLOOD SUGAR GOALS IN PREGNANCY

Before breakfast	60–90 mg/dl
Before lunch, supper, and bedtime snacks	60–105 mg/dl
After meals	less than 140 mg/dl
2 A.M. to 6 A.M.	60–100 mg/dl

RISKS OF DIABETES DURING PREGNANCY

- Increased risk of miscarriage
- Increased risk of birth defects; small skin discolorations, webbed toe, heart abnormalities, spina bifida, cleft lip, and cleft palate
- Increased risk of macrosomia (an abnormally large baby)

What is important to keep in mind is that the risks and complications can be negligible if you control your diabetes. If you have diabetes and you plan to get pregnant, you should get those blood sugars under good control before conception. You will need to measure your blood sugars frequently to achieve your goal. This discipline and perseverance will help you deal with motherhood after delivery. By working with your doctor and his or her team, you can maximize your chances, and your baby's chances, of having a great pregnancy without complications. You can do it!

DIABETES IS A MAJOR HEALTH PROBLEM AMONG HISPANICS

- Approximately one in every ten Hispanic adults has diabetes.
- Nearly 10 percent of Cuban Americans and Mexican Americans have diabetes.
- On average Latinos are nearly twice as likely to have diabetes as non-Hispanic whites.
- Approximately 25 percent of Mexican Americans and Puerto Ricans between the ages of forty-five and seventy-four have diabetes, and about 16 percent of Cuban Americans in this age-group have diabetes.
- Population studies among Hispanic women with diabetes show significantly higher death rates and complications during pregnancy.
- About one-third of total diabetes cases among Latinos twenty years old and older are undiagnosed.

PREECLAMPSIA OR TOXEMIA

Preeclampsia occurs in the last trimester of pregnancy. Its cause is unknown. Symptoms include blood pressure of 140 over 90, excessive weight gain, the presence of proteins in the urine, and fluid retention (with inflammation of the hands, ankles, and feet). High blood pressure is especially dangerous, and in severe cases it may cause seizures or other problems. Sometimes it is necessary to induce labor or to perform a cesarean even before the pregnancy reaches full term.

VAGINAL BLEEDING

If vaginal bleeding occurs prior to week twenty-eight, it could be a warning of impending abortion. After that stage, it could mean that the placenta (which is what is keeping the baby alive) is bleeding. If that is the case, your doctor will surely perform tests to verify the position of the placenta. **But regardless of when it occurs, if you have vaginal bleeding call your doctor immediately.**

MOTHERS WITH RH NEGATIVE (see Chapter 2, Blood Incompatibility)

If you belong to the 15 percent of the population that has Rh-negative blood, you would have problems only if you gave birth to an Rh-positive baby. These risks are minimal in the first pregnancy. However, you should receive an injection of anti-Rh immunoglobin in order to prevent any complications with future pregnancies.

STATISTICS ON RISKS

- Male embryos, fetuses, and babies run a greater risk of disease than females.
- In the United States, the risk for a woman having to have a cesarean birth is 21.1 percent (on the average). The probability of this increases with age, to 35 percent for pregnant women thirty-five or older.
- For a pregnant woman of twenty, the risk of her baby being born with Down's syndrome is 1 in 10,000. For a woman of forty-four, the risk increases to 1 in 38.
- Certain studies suggest that men who are exposed to toxic chemicals at work (like anesthesiologists, jet pilots, and deep-sea divers) have a higher probability of having male children than female.
- The national rate of infant mortality (from birth through the first year) is 10.1 deaths for every 1,000 live births in the United States.

PRENATAL TESTS

Medical advances allow us to determine whether the baby suffers from certain genetic problems before birth. These tests are recommended for women who suspect that they may run the greatest risk of having babies with problems.

AMNIOCENTESIS

Amniocentesis is almost always done between the fifteenth and the eighteenth week in order to determine whether there are abnormalities in the chromosomes (as in the case with

Down's syndrome) and/or in the development of the fetus (as in the case of malformations of the central nervous system). If there are serious problems with the baby, the parents have

the option of interrupting the pregnancy at that time. The test consists of the insertion through the abdomen of a very delicate needle that penetrates the amniotic fluid and extracts an ounce of the liquid surrounding the fetus. (Refer to the diagram.) The liquid is studied in the laboratory, and it takes from three to four weeks to obtain the information. Even though it is not painful, it can be uncomfortable. The risks are minimal and include, among others, bleeding, infection, and, in 1 out of 200 women, the risk of miscarriage.

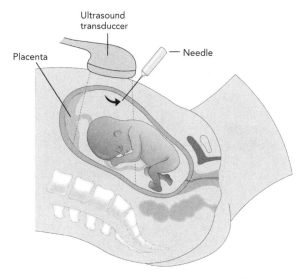

Ultrasound
transduccer

Needle

Placenta

Amniocentesis

INDICATIONS FOR AMNIOCENTESIS

- Being thirty-five years of age or older
- Having had a baby with a birth defect
- Having a birth defect
- Having a family history of birth defects
- Having a partner with a birth defect
- Having diabetes in certain women

ULTRASOUND

Ultrasound is painless and takes just a few minutes. It can be done at any stage of pregnancy. It's done by having the doctor or technician move the transducer across the woman's lower abdomen. Pictures can also be obtained by introducing the transducer into the vagina.

"We would love to know whether it's a girl or a boy. Is it possible to find this out with any certainty by means of an ultrasound?"

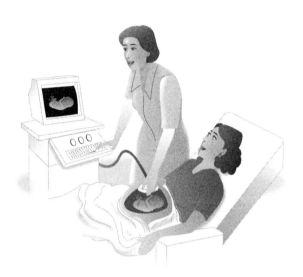

Ultrasound

Even though it's not one of the indications for the performance of an ultrasound, when the procedure is done for other reasons, the test can often tell you whether it is a boy or a girl. However, it is not 100 percent accurate. If you manage to see that it's a boy, you can tell it's a boy. But if you can't make out the penis, it might be a girl, or simply a boy who had his leg or another part of his body covering the genitals at the time of the ultrasound. However, amniocentesis, if required for other reasons, is very precise in determining the sex of the baby.

ULTRASOUND

The ultrasound uses high-frequency sound waves to create pictures of the fetus either in motion, on a TV monitor, or in still frames, using a camera. It works by sending out sound waves with a transducer (small handheld device); those sound waves bounce off the fetus and create an image.

REASONS FOR DOING AN ULTRASOUND

The purpose of the ultrasound may vary at different stages of the pregnancy. They include:

- Determining the age and size of the fetus
- Determining fetal position, movement, breathing, and heart rate
- Determining the due date
- Assisting with procedures like amniocentesis
- Determining the amount of amniotic fluid
- Determining the location of the placenta
- Determining certain abnormalities (i.e., birth defects, placental abnormalities, uterine abnormalities, etc.)
- Determining the number of fetuses

CHORIONIC VILLUS SAMPLING

This test also detects abnormalities in the chromosomes as well as the presence of certain hereditary genetic diseases. It is done by inserting a small tube through the cervix, via the vagina, and using it to extract a small piece of the placenta tissue. If the sample is obtained during the first attempt, the procedure takes only a few minutes. But, sometimes it is necessary to insert the catheter several times in order to obtain the tissue. Advantages over amniocentesis are that it can be done between the ninth and eleventh weeks, and that the results can be obtained in less than a week. Disadvantages are that it tends to be painful for some women and is less precise than the amniocentesis. In addition, there is a slightly higher risk of abortion.

TESTING THE MOTHER'S BLOOD FOR ALPHA-FETOPROTEIN

This test detects the level of alpha-fetoprotein in the mother's blood. Alpha-fetoprotein is abbreviated as AFP and is a substance produced by the fetus. A high level may indicate problems as serious as spina bifida (a congenital defect in which part of one or more vertebrae fail to develop completely, leaving a portion of the spinal cord exposed) or anencephaly (absence at birth of the brain, top of the skull, and spinal cord), or something as simple as the presence of twins. If it is low, it might indicate a chromosomal deficiency such as Down's syndrome. Only one to two of every fifty women who show a high level of alpha-fetoprotein in the initial reading run a risk that the fetus might be affected.

RISK DUE TO LACK OF PRENATAL CARE

Babies born to mothers who did not receive prenatal care have a three times higher risk of dying during the first year of life than babies born to mothers who received thorough medical attention.

The world's record for the oldest pregnant woman belongs to an Italian, Rossana Della Corte, who in July 1994, at age sixty-three, gave birth to a son.

PROTECTING YOUR BABY

VICES AND HABITS

Alcohol

Alcohol abuse may seriously affect the development of the fetus. Since it is not certain what amount of alcohol may be damaging, it's best to avoid alcoholic beverages during pregnancy.

If you have problems with alcoholism, seek help immediately (ideally before becoming pregnant). You can call Alcoholics Anonymous in your area or ask your physician for help. If you are already pregnant, remember that whenever you get drunk, the fetus experiences the same effects. If alcohol can cause liver damage in an adult, imagine the damage that can be done to a tiny baby whose organs, including the brain, are just forming. The damage may be irreversible and could include mental retardation.

FETAL ALCOHOL SYNDROME

Of all the causes of birth defects, the syndrome resulting from exposure of the fetus to alcohol is the one that is easiest to prevent.

If you are pregnant, refuse alcoholic beverages. Reserve the celebrations with alcohol for after the pregnancy and when you have stopped breast-feeding. If you have problems with alcoholism, consult your doctor. Doing so is not a sign of weakness; it's a sign of responsibility.

A SOBER PREGNANCY

One group of physicians who consider that even small quantities of alcohol imbibed during pregnancy may affect fetal development protested a book that guaranteed there was no danger in drinking a glass of wine a day during pregnancy. Recent investigation done at the University of Pittsburgh showed that several of the newborns of mothers who drank less than one glass of alcoholic beverages per day during their pregnancy weighed less, were shorter, and had a lower IQ (intelligence quotient) than is considered average. According to Dr. Patti Munter, the executive director of the National Organization of Fetal-Alcohol Syndrome, the statements in the book *Your Health: Two Doctors Explore the Health Benefits of Wine*—written by Drs. David Whitten and Martin Lipp—could cause irreparable damage to millions of children.

Drugs

Mothers who use drugs during pregnancy put their health and the health of their babies at risk. Babies of mothers addicted to cocaine or "crack," for example, are born with that addiction and plagued by terrible health problems and irreparable birth defects, perhaps even the lack of a brain.

As far as the pregnant woman is concerned, there is no "strong drug" or "mild drug"; any drug is harmful to her and to her baby. Marijuana, which many mistakenly consider harmless, can cause the baby to have cardiac and cerebral disorders.

If you are pregnant, say no to all drugs.

DRUGS AND PREGNANCY

- Fifteen percent of women of childbearing age (between fifteen and forty-four years old) in the United States abuse addictive substances. Of those, 44 percent have tried marijuana and 14 percent have used cocaine at least once during their pregnancy.
- It is estimated that 375,000 babies in the United States are exposed to harmful drugs every year. This is due to the fact that 1 out of every 10 mothers has taken illegal drugs.
- Women who use cocaine during the first months of pregnancy run a five times greater risk of their babies developing urinary tract defects.
- Medical attention in the United States for a baby addicted to crack, resulting from exposure during pregnancy, costs around $100,000 during the first three months of life.

Smoking

Even though you have seen celebrities like Melanie Griffith smoke during pregnancy, don't follow her example. Smoking reduces the amount of oxygen the baby needs for normal development and increases the amount of carbon dioxide, nicotine, and tar in your bloodstream. It is also passed along to your baby. Babies of mothers who smoke are born smaller and have a greater chance of premature birth. Smoking also increases the possibility of abortion, congenital malformations, and death of babies following their birth.

SAY NO TO CIGARETTE SMOKE
(AND TO CIGARS AND PIPES AS WELL)

The majority of future mothers know that smoking during pregnancy is dangerous for the baby they're expecting, but new research assures us that being around someone who is smoking is also dangerous. It has been proven that the inhaled cigarette smoke of others also reaches the fetus through the mother's bloodstream, and following the birth, the baby inhales the secondhand smoke directly. There are studies that show the presence of a disintegrated form of nicotine in the hair and bloodstream of mothers and newborns exposed to other people's cigarette smoke.

It is almost as important that your partner not smoke as well. Exposure to secondhand cigarette smoke may also affect you and your baby.

Ideally, you will stop smoking before becoming pregnant, but if you haven't done so, it's never too late. Try again. A good mental exercise that will help you give up smoking is to imagine that your baby is smoking and inhaling all of your smoke. Some pregnant women have resorted to methods such as hypnosis, acupuncture, or a nicotine patch, but if you decide on these, it is essential that you consult your doctor first.

Don't think that once the baby is born he or she won't be affected by your smoking. During the breast-feeding period, cigarettes continue to be dangerous, since nicotine is transferred from the mother's blood through the milk. Besides, your cigarette smoke, or that of your partner, may increase the risk of respiratory illnesses in the infant.

Medicines

During your pregnancy, the only medicines you should be taking are those prescribed by your doctor, or those that you used to take and that have been approved by him or her. The ingredients of the medicines you take—like everything you ingest—could penetrate the placenta, in which the case the fetus is ingesting it too.

For common discomforts of pregnancy (dizziness, nausea, pains, constipation, anxiety, insomnia, nervousness), try to use natural remedies approved by your doctor, not medicines.

DANGEROUS MEDICINE

A University of Michigan researcher warned that a common medicine containing ACE inhibitors, if taken by pregnant women to control high blood pressure, may cause considerable damage to the kidneys of newborns. This doesn't mean that if you had high blood pressure before, or during, your pregnancy, you shouldn't take your medicine. What it does mean is that, if you are planning on becoming pregnant and are taking medicine for high blood pressure (or any other medical problem), you should consult your doctor so that he or she can change your medicine to one that does not affect the baby (such as methyldopate in the case of high blood pressure). Don't stop taking any medicine prescribed by your doctor without consulting him or her beforehand. This could also be dangerous.

If you consult your doctor about any problem, he or she can prescribe medicines that will not affect your baby. Always follow the instructions. Don't take any more than the amount indicated.

Regarding medicines that are sold over-the-counter without a prescription—don't take anything without consulting your doctor. Even though you think a medicine as common as aspirin is not harmful, it may be during pregnancy.

If you have a problem like hypertension or diabetes, or if you are taking any medicine on a regular basis, it is ideal to consult your doctor when you are planning on getting pregnant. If you are already pregnant, consult your doctor immediately. There are medicines that should not be stopped all of a sudden. Your doctor might substitute them with others that either pose no risk, or pose fewer risks to your baby.

Caffeine

Some studies have found a correlation between the excess of caffeine and birth defects. Nevertheless, more recent studies with the equivalent of two to three cups of coffee a day don't seem to corroborate that. The Food and Drug Administration (FDA) has adopted a conservative stance on the subject. They recommend that, if a pregnant woman wants to consume drinks or foods containing caffeine, she should avoid ingesting more than the equivalent of three cups of coffee a day.

Some doctors recommend that the pregnant woman substitute those products containing caffeine (like coffee, *mate,* and some soft drinks and teas) with similar decaffeinated beverages, or with natural fruit juices or mineral water.

If you are in the habit of drinking coffee and you decide that you want to stop, because it is a stimulant, you might notice a change in your energy level at first, but it's only for a short while. Exercising more and eating small quantities of food more frequently will help you maintain your accustomed level of energy.

JUST ONE CUP, PLEASE

The American Medical Association reports that moderate use of caffeine by pregnant women does not increase the risk of miscarriage. According to a study done by Dr. James L. Mills and his colleagues at the National Institutes of Health, no evidence was found proving that moderate use of caffeine (no more than three cups per day) increases the risk of miscarriage or causes a delay in intrauterine growth, or microcephaly (small head) in the fetuses of pregnant women. **But be careful! Three cups of American coffee are equivalent to one little cup of Cuban coffee or espresso.**

And remember that *mate* contains caffeine too.

ENVIRONMENTAL FACTORS
Pets

Since cats can transmit a parasite known as *Toxoplasma gondii,* which can cause an infection (toxoplasmosis) in the mother, and that infection can cause a miscarriage or harm the baby during the pregnancy, it is recommended that you always wash your hands after playing with a cat. You should thoroughly wash all areas frequented by the cat and use gloves every time you clean the litter box (since the parasite may be found in cat feces). These instructions should be followed even if your cat is extremely clean and well groomed.

Toxoplasma is also found in raw meat. Take the same precautions in the kitchen when you prepare it, and ensure that meat has been well cooked before eating it.

Household accidents

Despite carrying around a belly weighing several additional pounds, and despite feeling more exhausted and less agile than usual, many women believe that they can keep on behaving as if they were athletes at home (and outside).

PAY ATTENTION TO THE ENVIRONMENT

A report from Yale University indicates that women who live near toxic waste sites have a greater chance of giving birth to children with birth defects. Even though this has been suspected for some time, this study is the first to offer concrete proof of this relationship.

In the first place, keep in mind that your body's equilibrium is different now, since your center of gravity is propelling you forward. The joints (above all the knees and ankles) are slightly weaker than usual, which increases the likelihood of falling. Even though it is slight, a certain risk exists with any fall taken by a pregnant woman, especially if she falls forward.

For this reason, if you fall—even if you feel fine and don't think you've hurt yourself—you should tell your doctor; he or she will decide whether it's necessary to perform any tests.

Fatigue can decrease your stability and your emotional and psychological state (e.g., worries about the pregnancy, etc.) and can take your attention away from what you are doing.

Fortunately, the baby inside you is quite protected by nature itself. The baby is surrounded by an efficient protective system—amniotic fluid, membranes, muscular fibers of the uterus, and even the bones and muscles of the abdominal and pelvic cavity—which absorbs bruises and movements. This does not mean that deep bruises and lesions can't have a disastrous impact on you and your baby. If this is the case, you will notice it by means of vaginal bleeding, pain in the abdomen, uterine contractions, or the leakage of amniotic fluid.

In some cases, excessive activity on the part of the fetus following an accident might be a sign that the baby has suffered a concussion. In these cases, it is essential to advise your doctor immediately or go to an emergency room right away.

Even if you are a very fastidious person, this is a time when you should accept the fact that certain household tasks are more important than others. It is important to accept that, in your condition, you might not be able to dedicate the same time and energy as usual to taking care of your home. Someone (either a family member or a temporary helper) can assist you with cleaning, or you can buy the washer and/or dryer you've always dreamed of (something that will be very useful after the arrival of the baby, anyway).

A FULL-TIME JOB

Pregnancy is a twenty-four-hour-a-day job for nine months. Remember that, in case you feel tired.

PREPARING YOUR HOME

Around week thirty-six, if you work outside the home, you should be enjoying your maternity leave from work, and this is the ideal time—unless you are confined to total bed rest, or you feel too tired—to dedicate yourself to the task of preparing your home for the baby's arrival. Here is some basic advice:

- Accept the help of a friend, your partner, or a family member to put everything in order, and to see that you don't take on the entire task of the preparation yourself.
- Remember, while cleaning the house and decorating you shouldn't move furniture or carry heavy objects; these activities could cause problems or, at the very least, a premature birth.
- Fill your refrigerator with food that's easy to prepare, or that can be frozen, such as breads and vegetables.
- Buy things like toilet paper, detergent, diapers, cleaning supplies, and things that will be useful in the home when, after the birth, you have less time to go to the market.

- Dedicate one room in the house, if possible, solely to your newborn, although this is not absolutely necessary (especially when you consider that many mothers want to have their baby's crib in their room for the first few months).
- If you can, dedicate a room in your house for everything related to the baby—a place that, in addition to being a bedroom, can serve as a playroom, as a nap room, and as a dining room, bathroom, and dressing room.

MYRKA DELLANOS
Broadcast journalist and hostess of *Exclusively with Myrka Dellanos*

My only daughter, Alexa Carolina, was born on December 30, 1993. The worst experience of my pregnancy was the morning sickness, which lasted five months. I did everything I was told (crackers, syrups) and nothing.... I lost weight because all I could eat was cereal and grapefruit juice. I felt so ill when I got home from work that I would bathe, throw myself on the bed, and say, "Dear God, please let me sleep so that I won't feel so sick."

But after the first five months, I felt fine. I ate everything, I looked good, and emotionally, I felt fabulous. Definitely, the fifth to the eighth months of pregnancy were the best.

I learned from my pregnancy that the best thing is to keep as busy as possible. I worked until the last day, and my water broke during an interview! Even though you may not feel great, working makes time go by faster.

What I plan to do the next time I get pregnant is to exercise more. I swam and walked quite a lot, but I could have done more. The more active you are when you're pregnant, the better everything goes. The delivery is easier, you're healthier, you don't gain so much weight, and you feel better all around. For my next one, I plan to continue weightlifting (naturally, under the supervision of my trainer and my doctor), doing aerobics, and walking as much as possible. My best advice to first timers is that, if they are eating healthily and doing some type of exercise, they don't need to worry about gaining too much weight. When I got to the eighth month and saw such a huge stomach, I thought I'd never look the same again. Enjoy your pregnancy because it is a beautiful moment in a woman's life and, though it may seem long, it only lasts nine months.

Chapter 4

WEIGHT, DIET, AND EXERCISE

WEIGHT ISSUES DURING PREGNANCY

If you are overweight, it's a good idea to lose weight before getting pregnant, since weight-loss diets are not recommended during pregnancy.

Don't think that, just because you are "eating for two" or for "one and a half," you now have permission to reach a disproportionate weight. According to the American College of Obstetricians and Gynecologists, a pregnant woman should gain only between twenty-five and thirty-five pounds during the nine-month period. If the woman is very thin at the onset of pregnancy, she may be able to gain up to forty pounds.

The majority of women worry about their weight during pregnancy—whether they are gaining too much, or not enough. That's why it is important to consult your doctor regarding your particular case—as to how much you should gain, and over what period of time.

Weigh yourself each week. Ideally, your weight gain should be gradual. It is estimated that women gain around ten pounds in the first twenty weeks, and one pound every week thereafter. When you don't eat enough, or when you eat poorly and there are insufficient nutrients, the baby might experience more problems at birth.

It is preferable to try not to gain too much weight until the fourth month since, up until this time, weight gain is due to the accumulation of fluid and fat in the maternal tissues. After the fifth month, weight gain is due to the increase in weight inside the uterus, the placenta, the amniotic fluid, and the baby itself.

DISTRIBUTION OF WEIGHT GAIN FOR A FULL-TERM PREGNANCY

Uterus	2 pounds
Placenta	1½ pounds
Amniotic Fluid	2 pounds
Baby	6 to 8 pounds
Fat, fluid, etc., within the mother	4 to 6 pounds

ABOUT NUTRITION

Remember that what you eat is what is feeding your baby. So maintaining a healthy and balanced diet is especially important now. The number of calories you consume each day should be increased by 300 to 500, if you were not overweight prior to becoming pregnant. This will vary somewhat, depending on how active you are. But your doctor might recommend 800 additional calories per day if you are underweight, or less than 300 extra calories per day if you are overweight. He or she will also advise you on the amount and the nutritional content of the food you eat.

If the mother-to-be follows a diet that is healthy and complete, if she exercises and reduces stress during the nine months of pregnancy, she will increase the possibility that her child will be born in excellent health. Obviously, maintaining healthy habits before getting pregnant is ideal, therefore making the changes less drastic during the nine months of pregnancy.

Along with the healthy habits of everyday life, we have already spoken about caffeine, alcohol, and drugs in Chapter 3. Here are some additional recommendations:

MYTH: THE FIRST CHILD ALWAYS ARRIVES LATE

Although the first child is frequently born a little after the projected due date, this is not always the case. The timing of the birth varies from woman to woman, and sometimes from pregnancy to pregnancy in the same woman. Actually it can be linked in a closer way to the length of the menstrual period. If you tend to have your period every thirty days, it's possible that you might give birth a little later than if you have your period every twenty-seven days.

PLANNING YOUR DIET

- Try to eat more or less at the same time every day in an unhurried, stress-free environment. Due to the growth of the womb, many pregnant women find that eating small amounts several times a day works best for them.
- Don't think that, because you ate too much one day, you should fast the next; this is not good for a pregnant woman, as her ideal diet should be regular and constant.
- Prepare simple meals, with few sauces, condiments, and seasoning.
- The best way to eat meat and fish is baked, broiled, or grilled. Use natural seasonings such as lemon, virgin olive oil, a little salt, and herbs such as laurel, cumin, parsley, sweet basil, and pepper.

IN GENERAL

- Eat slowly and carefully chew all your food.
- Variety and quality are especially important.
- Don't use your pregnancy as an excuse to overeat and gain too much weight.
- Don't undereat; this could endanger your baby's chance of survival early in pregnancy and could result in a small baby.

VEGETABLES

- Include at least a cup of leafy green vegetables in your daily diet, either at lunch or at dinner. Some of these are broccoli, spinach, watercress, asparagus, lettuce, green pepper, etc. They all contain three elements that you really need: vitamin A, vitamin C, and folic acid.

- Don't leave out other popular vegetables such as beets, avocados, cabbage, carrots, cauliflower, corn, tomatoes, etc. These should be eaten *in addition to* the leafy green ones.

- Try to eat as many of your vegetables raw as you can (after thoroughly washing and scrubbing them) because they contain more nutrients. Many times, when cooking vegetables, we place them in water and heat them to such a degree that we eliminate their nutritional properties. However, if your stomach is incapable of digesting raw veggies, try to steam or boil them in just a little water, and instead of throwing that water out, use it as a base for soup or puree. That water is full of nutrients!

FOLIC ACID

According to the U.S. Department of Health Services, all women of childbearing age should increase their consumption of folic acid as a means of preventing birth defects in their children. It is believed that a deficiency in folic acid—a type of vitamin B found in fruits, green vegetables, beans, and grains—is related to neurological defects such as spina bifida and anencephaly. It has been recommended that women take 1 milligram of folic acid a day, which is the amount in prenatal vitamins, although many pregnant women can take more than that amount since, frequently, their regular diet does not contain enough folic acid.

FRUITS

- Don't forget your fruit! Eat at least two items of fruit per day (well washed). Again, it is preferable to eat them raw, for the same reasons as above.

CARBOHYDRATES (SUGARS)

- Be sure to include a good dose of complex carbohydrates, several of which should have a high fiber content. The pregnant woman's diet is not complete without them.
- Don't forget to include some of the following in each meal: lentils, milk, pastas, rice, sweet potatoes, corn tortillas, soybeans, breakfast cereals (oats, barley), whole grain wheat or rye bread, etc.
- Include other foods rich in carbohydrates, such as lettuce, celery, cabbage, artichokes, potatoes, carrots, beets, and most fruits.

EAT TWO OR MORE SERVINGS OF FRUITS A DAY

One serving of fruits is equivalent to:

1 medium apple, pear, banana

2 medium plums or apricots

½ cup berries, cantaloupe, pineapple, fruit cocktail

¾ cup of fruit juice

EAT TWO OR MORE SERVINGS OF VEGETABLES A DAY

One serving of vegetables is equivalent to:

½ cup broccoli, carrots, green beans, zucchini, bell peppers, spinach, peas, corn

½ cup vegetable juice

1 medium potato, sweet potato

½ medium avocado

½ cup raw lettuce, green salad, cabbage

½ cup tomato sauce

EAT SEVEN OR MORE SERVINGS
OF BREAD AND CEREALS A DAY

One serving is equivalent to:

1 slice of whole grain or enriched bread	½ bagel
1 cup dry cereal	1¼-inch pancake or 4-inch waffle
1 corn or flour tortilla	1 muffin or biscuit
½ cup oatmeal or grits	½ cup rice or pasta
5 crackers	1 whole wheat pita
½ cup granola	½ hamburger or hot dog bun

FATS

- Don't avoid all fats! Even though you might not believe this, fats, in moderation, are good for pregnant women! These substances are rich in vitamins A and D and provide a lot of the energy that is so necessary at the time of birth. But don't get too used to them because, after you give birth, you are going to have to noticeably reduce their consumption if you want to wear the clothes you wore before you got pregnant.
- Avoid excess fats in general, but especially saturated fats, like animal fats, which tend to increase cholesterol levels in the blood.
- Avoid fried foods, canned foods, and creamy foods. It is preferable to eat fats that come from natural foods such as avocado and shrimp and to use vegetable oil (olive oil, for example). If you eat meat, discard the fatty portions. That way you will receive greater benefits with fewer calories.

PROTEINS

- Eat one food that is rich in protein every day such as red meat, poultry, eggs, fish, cheese, vegetables, beans, lentils, or garbanzos. Proteins are important for muscle formation.

EAT TWO OR MORE SERVINGS
OF MEAT OR MEAT ALTERNATIVES A DAY

One serving is equivalent to:

3 ounces chicken, fish, turkey	1 cup tofu
1 cup dried, baked, or refried beans	½ cup nuts
3 slices lunch meat	3 ounces hamburger, steak
1 cup cooked lentils, or in soup	4 tablespoons peanut butter
3 ounces ham, lean beef, veal, lamb, or pork	2 ounces frankfurters
	3 ounces spare ribs or sausage

Remember, it is healthier to avoid fried and greasy foods. This is especially important if you do not want to gain too much weight.

LIQUIDS

- Drink milk during pregnancy to help ensure your baby will have healthy bones and teeth. Consuming four servings of milk or milk products is recommended on a daily basis throughout your pregnancy. If you don't like milk, you can replace it with yogurt, cheese, or ice cream. If you can't digest milk products, look for those that are labeled "lactose reduced." Calcium intake is extremely important. A minimum of 1,000 milligrams daily is recommended to protect the mother's teeth and prevent toxemia. If you cannot tolerate milk, take calcium supplements.
- Drink between six and eight glasses of water a day (a good recommendation for all of us). This is something that pregnant women can't overdo. If you don't like water very much, sweeten it with a bit of vegetable or fruit juice.

CANNED FOODS

- Avoid eating canned foods as much as possible, although it is convenient to have some canned food items at home when you feel very tired, or in preparation for the days following the pregnancy. Many of these packaged foods contain substances (preservatives, etc.) that are not exactly healthy.

- Also avoid frozen foods, the majority of which contain a variety of additives and chemicals.

CONSUME FOUR OR MORE SERVINGS OF MILK OR OTHER DAIRY PRODUCTS A DAY

One serving is equivalent to:

1 cup milk, buttermilk, plain yogurt

1 cup tofu fortified soy milk

1½ ounces (2 slices) mozzarella cheese, low-fat cheese

¾ cup cottage cheese, frozen yogurt, ice cream

These can be nonfat or low-fat

FOODS TO AVOID

- Those that you know make you gain weight easily
- Excessively sweetened foods, sugary desserts, and pastries
- Highly salty foods
- Raw eggs, raw fish, or raw meat
- Freshwater shellfish (due to the risk of insecticide contamination)
- Tap water that hasn't been boiled, if you live in an area where the drinking water might be contaminated
- Excessive soft drinks, coffee, tea, or caffeinated colas

Every year there are some 40,000 babies born to women between the ages of forty and forty-nine in the United States; 38,000 of those babies are born to mothers between the ages of forty and forty-four, while the rest (some 2,000) are born to mothers between the ages of forty-five and forty-nine.

VITAMINS AND MINERALS
FOR THE PREGNANT WOMAN

A balanced diet should provide you with most of the vitamins and minerals required by your body and the baby you are carrying inside you. Nevertheless, your doctor will likely recommend a prenatal supplement that includes iron. Sometimes it is difficult to get enough iron from the foods you eat.

VITAMINS

The following are the essential vitamins that should be included in the pregnant woman's diet. Look for foods that contain them, and make them a basic part of your everyday diet. If some of them aren't your favorites, try to eat them once in a while anyway. Remember that it's only nine months, and a balanced diet is essential for your baby to be born healthy.

Vitamin A

Whole milk, cheese, egg yolks, liver, vegetables

Vitamin B_1

Liver and other animal organs, pork, legumes, dried fruit, potatoes, oranges, grapefruit, pineapple, egg whites

Vitamin B_2

Kidneys, liver, whole milk, cheese, dried fruit, beans

Vitamin B_3

Whole milk, egg yolk, beef, poultry, fish, whole grain bread, brown rice, mushrooms, tomatoes

Vitamin B_{12}

Whole milk, liver, egg yolks

Vitamin C

Whole milk, eggs, fish, fruit, especially citrus fruits

Vitamin D

Liver, eggs, fish, butter

Vitamin E

Found in almost all the foods mentioned above, and in many more

Vitamin K

Spinach, tomatoes, cabbage, egg yolks

Folic acid

Green leafy vegetables, liver, dried fruit

Niacin

Poultry, fish, liver, dried fruit

MINERALS

Our body can't survive without minerals, and the same goes for the baby you are carrying in your womb. For example, iron is essential for the formation of blood, calcium is integral to bone development, and without sodium and potassium, the body's liquids can't constantly renew themselves. The following should not be absent from your diet:

Calcium

Milk, cheese, vegetables such as broccoli and spinach

Phosphorus

Fish, meat, eggs, milk, vegetables

Iron

Meat, liver, animal organs and bones, potatoes, lentils, beans, broccoli, spinach, asparagus, mushrooms, peaches, figs, grapes

Potassium

Contained in a great majority of foods

Sodium

Found in almost every food item, especially in salt (you obtain an adequate amount from the salt you use for cooking)

Iodine

Fish, vegetables (especially asparagus, mushrooms, and carrots)

TEN SUGGESTIONS FOR A HEALTHY DIET

1. A balanced diet doesn't just guarantee the normal and healthy development of your baby, it also helps you avoid common digestive problems experienced during pregnancy, like nausea and excess stomach acid.
2. If your bouts of nausea last longer than the first trimester, try to eat small meals several times a day, which is better than heavy meals followed by a prolonged period without eating.
3. Avoid excessive consumption of salt and condiments.
4. Try to cook simple meals in order to obtain the maximum amount of nutrients, which can be lost as a result of long cooking times.
5. It is not advisable to boil vegetables that could be eaten raw; boiling robs them of their vitamins and minerals, which get dissolved in the water. For those that require cooking, buy a vegetable steamer.
6. Get used to eating broiled meat and fish, and avoid fried foods. The oils used in frying digest more slowly and, besides increasing calories (if you are watching your weight), they can be more difficult to digest.
7. To improve the taste of food, use lemon, olive oil, and aromatic herbs for seasoning.
8. Eggs are a wonderful food for pregnant women, as long as they are cooked and not fried. You should never eat them raw, in order to avoid the possibility of contamination by bacteria such as *Salmonella*. If you prefer to eat them in omelet form, don't deprive yourself of this, but use vegetable oil instead of lard. Because of the amount of cholesterol in the yolk, limit your egg intake to a maximum of four a week.
9. If you suffer from heartburn or excess stomach acid, you will have to suppress your taste for rich sauces and fried foods, unless you want to suffer the consequences.

10. As for sweets, try to eat fruit instead of pastries and other foods that contain refined sugar. This will not only help you control your weight, but it will also provide you with vitamins, minerals, and fiber that you and your baby both need. At the same time, you will be using the best remedy to fight constipation, a common malady during pregnancy.

In spite of all the above, this does not mean that you have to sacrifice all of your favorite foods. I don't mean to say that you can't enjoy *tamales, mole, enchiladas, quesadillas,* or *buñuelos* **once in a while**, if you like Mexican food. Or *empanadas* and *churrasco* with *chimichurri,* if you like Argentine food. Or *pupusas,* if you like Salvadoran fare. If Puerto Rican food is your thing, you might want to eat *mofongo, bacalaitos fritos* (fried cod), roast pork, *empanadas de jueyes, adobo,* and *churros* **from time to time**. If you are of Cuban descent, your mouth might water at the mere mention of roast pork. Cuban food also has its share of fried items, such as *tostones* and *maduros,* fried yuca, *choripán,* sandwiches, and *ropa vieja,* all of which you can enjoy **in moderation**. Since they are all high in fats, you should consider eating a small portion of any of them two to three times a month maximum.

SOME SUGGESTIONS FOR EATING OUT

- You should order grilled chicken, fish, or meat, without the sauce, or with the sauce on the side. That way you control the amount you put on.
- The same applies to salads. The dressing might be just lemon or balsamic vinegar, with or without a bit of olive oil, or some other type of dressing on the side, so you can control the amount.
- If you're going to eat pasta, it's best to order pasta with a tomato sauce instead of a cream or cheese sauce. Remember that the amount is important. If you eat pasta, don't eat bread, rice, or potatoes at the same meal. Of course, a baked potato is very healthy, especially if you eat it with nonfat or low-fat sour cream (or even better, plain nonfat yogurt), but avoid bacon.
- Raw or steamed vegetables without sauces, or with the sauce on the side, add fiber, in addition to vitamins and excellent nutritional value.
- Fruit can be eaten in between meals, as a main course, or for dessert. Again, fruits are rich in fiber, vitamins, and nutritional value.

- Remember that it's important to include proteins in your diet. If you like salads, you can always order one with cottage cheese, with plain yogurt, or with chicken, turkey or egg.
- If you like spicy sauces, garlic, or onion, and they don't cause you to experience digestive problems, go ahead and enjoy them.
- Avoid foods that are too greasy, especially those that contain lard instead of vegetable or olive oil.

THE BENEFITS OF EXERCISE

Exercise is not only good for the pregnant woman and her baby, but it also makes delivery shorter and easier, reducing pain during delivery and helping with recovery. Moderate and regular exercise reduces the risk of diabetes during pregnancy, back pain, leg cramps, varicose veins, and constipation.

Women with a history of miscarriage, heart trouble, hemorrhages, or other problems, will be forbidden by their doctors from participating in most forms of exercise.

Which exercises are good for a pregnant woman depends in part on her physical condition and her exercise routine before becoming pregnant. In all cases, however, there comes a time during the pregnancy when she will have to avoid or reduce certain exercises. Even if she is in excellent physical shape, she should always consult with her doctor. Don't forget to pay attention to what your body is telling you. Avoid getting overheated and drink lots of liquids.

ONE PLAN FOR EATING OUT

If you go to a Mexican restaurant, order a shrimp cocktail or an appetizer salad (with *nopalitos*, for example) and fruit juice. That way, while the others eat the greasy *totopos* (or chips) with their tequilas, you can enjoy your salad (which you can order with warm tortillas) and your juice. Avoid refried beans, but you can order boiled beans or bean soup. Avoid tacos with fried tortillas, but enjoy tacos with soft, warm tortillas, or a burrito, or chicken fajitas.

Pending prior approval by your doctor, here are some general guidelines regarding exercise during pregnancy:

- Pulse rate should not exceed 140 beats per minute regardless of the exercise you choose to do.
- *Walk* until you reach a speed of three miles per hour. Walk every chance you can get, but never get overtired. Maintain a steady pace, but don't hurry. It is ideal to walk in areas far removed from traffic, where you are not subject to inhaling toxic fumes from cars.
- *Ride a bicycle,* but only until the second trimester (thereafter, continue at home on a stationary bike). On very steep hills, get off the bicycle and walk.
- *Aerobic exercise* is great, as long as it is low impact.
- *Swimming* is excellent (Imagine: for a time you won't feel the weight of your belly!); however, don't swim in very cold or in very hot water. Aerobic exercise in the pool is also beneficial, since water offers the muscles a natural and balanced resistance for the whole body.
- *Tennis, jogging, diving,* and similar sports should be indulged in during pregnancy only if you have always participated in them. However, it is recommended that you consult your doctor—often he or she will suggest that you reduce the frequency and, sometimes, suspend these activities altogether after the fifth month.
- *Yoga* exercises designed specifically for pregnant women have helped many feel better and have easier deliveries. They are recommended only under the supervision of an expert and as long as your doctor thinks that they pose no risk. Besides, yoga is excellent for controlling one's breathing.
- *Warm-up exercises* should be done first, and you should stop exercising as soon as you feel tired or you lack air. Stretching exercises, provided they are not done to excess, are very good.
- Avoid excessive exercise that overheats your body, just as you should avoid saunas and hot baths.
- After the fourth month, don't do exercises in which you have to lie on your back on the floor since this could decrease the flow of blood to the uterus.
- Stop any exercise if you experience hemorrhage, pain, dizziness, palpitations, shortness of breath, fainting, or other abnormal symptoms. Each body is different, and many women who are accustomed to exercising may be able to keep on doing so

without any problem until the advanced stages of their pregnancy. Since there is no rule, you should follow your doctor's advice and pay attention to what your body is telling you. If you feel tired or experience pain, don't try to overcome the situation with more exercise. Every time your body says, "Stop, I want to rest," pay attention immediately.

- **Track and field, weightlifting, tennis, horseback riding, jogging (running), and intense aerobic exercise are least recommended for pregnant women.**

DEVELOPING AN EXERCISE PROGRAM

WARM-UP EXERCISES

Before beginning your exercise session, you should prepare your body with brief warm-up movements, such as these:

- With your arms stretched out in front and your fingers extended, bend your hands at the wrist, first up, then down.

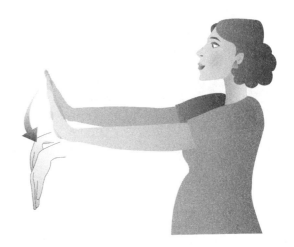

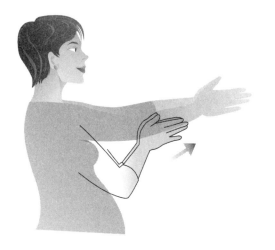

- Place your arms at chest level, with your hands touching, and stretch them out in front of you.

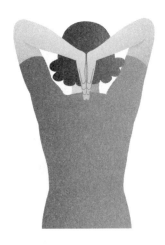

- Raise your arms out in back, toward the upper back, and try to make the palms of your hands touch.

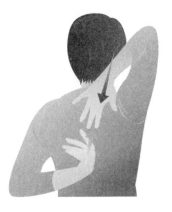

- Raise one arm, stretch it upward, and bend it in backward, in such a way that your hand is touching your back; lower the other arm and bend it in backward in such a way that the back of the hand touches the back; try to grab the fingers of one hand with the fingers of the other; reverse the position of both arms.

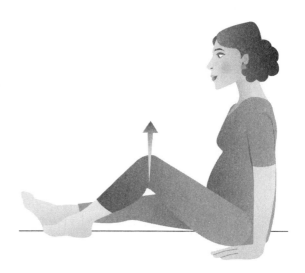

- While seated on the floor with your hands placed flat on the floor at your sides, stretch out your legs and alternately bend your knees, first one leg, then the other.

EXERCISES FOR THE PELVIS

These help prepare the body for the delivery and a speedier recovery. If you keep them up after the birth, they help you recover muscle tone and avoid problems such as urinary incontinence. Their advantage is that it's not necessary to go to a gym to do them; you can do them at any time.

Pelvic exercises tend to strengthen a series of muscles that support the intestines, the bladder, and the uterus. These muscles play an important role at the time of delivery and should, at that moment, be in the best possible physical condition. Try to do them while you are watching your favorite television show, seated in your car when you're at a stoplight, cleaning your house . . . and even when you're making love! You'll be surprised to find out that they'll also help you increase your sexual pleasure.

These exercises are even more important when you bear in mind that the muscles in the abdominal area and the pelvis soften and stretch during pregnancy. In addition, they are weakened by having to support the weight of the baby. One symptom of the loss of strength in these muscles is urinary incontinence, that is, the involuntary escape of a small amount of urine upon performing certain activities such as running, coughing, or even laughing boisterously.

That's why it's of the utmost importance to strengthen this muscle group with exercises such as these:

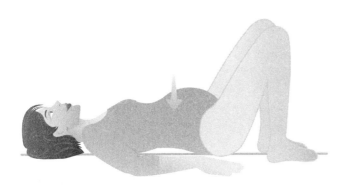

● Lie on your back face-up, with your knees bent, and the soles of the feet on the floor. Contract the muscles in the pelvic region as though you were trying to stop the flow of urine. Imagine that you are trying to make that little stream that wants to escape go back inside, by contracting and pulling those muscles in; relax the muscles every so often, but without letting go of the pressure, and then pull them back inside again. Do this exercise ten times in a row, at least three times a day, holding the final contraction of each series for a few seconds, then letting go slowly. You can even do this exercise seated, though, naturally, it's more thorough when you're lying down.

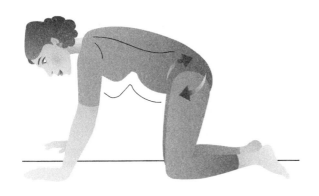

● Get down on all fours, with the palms of your hands and your knees on the floor, and your back as straight as possible. Either have someone seated beside you in the beginning, to correct your posture, or look at yourself in the mirror. Pull your abdominal (belly) muscles in, tightening your buttocks, and at the same time try to bring your pelvis forward. It is important to maintain steady rhythmic breathing, exhaling each time you bring the pelvis forward (and inhaling when you move it backward). Keep the pelvis as far forward as you can for several seconds (the back will curve lightly up), and then, after letting go of the air you were holding on to, bring your pelvis back to its initial position by the time you inhale. It's as though you were swinging the pelvis forward and backward like a pendulum. Do this at least three times a day.

EXERCISES FOR THE POSTURE

- Pregnant women frequently experience back pain, especially during the last months, because, at that stage, the fetus attains its greatest weight. Therefore, exercises that force you to straighten your back, either standing or lying down, will make you feel more comfortable and will relieve the cramps caused by the weight in your belly.

- Stand in front of a full-length mirror and correct your posture. Be conscious of always keeping your back straight—that way the baby's weight will be shared by your thighs, buttocks, and stomach. This will take part of the load off the back, decreasing pain in that area.

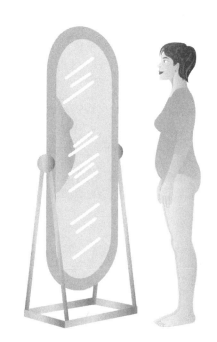

EXERCISES FOR THE LEGS

- Leg cramps are one of the most common problems in pregnant women; they happen mostly at night, making sleep difficult. They occur as a result of circulatory problems that can be alleviated with exercises to rotate the feet. These are so simple that you can do them seated, even while you're at the office. While sitting, bend your feet up toward you and gently stretch your legs. Then with your feet flexed toward you rotate them out, down, in, and up and reverse in, down, out, and up. Repeat these rotations three to five times.

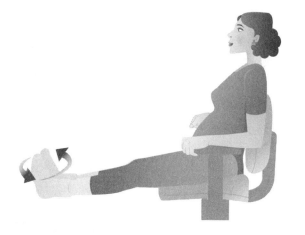

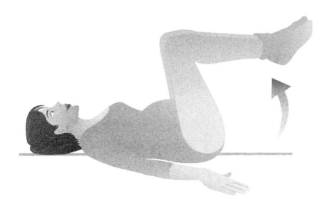

- Also to relieve leg cramps, raise the legs slowly while you are lying down, with knees bent and the soles of the feet planted on the floor or on the bed.

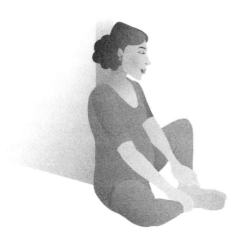

- To help make the thighs and pelvis more flexible, and to strengthen the back, sit on the floor on a soft surface (this will be easier if you place a cushion below each leg) and, with your back as straight as possible, bend your legs in, placing the feet sole to sole in front of the pelvis; you can help maintain this position by placing your hands on your ankles. If it is easier, support your back against a wall. Hold this position for a minute, or at least thirty seconds. Then relax the body for one or two minutes. Repeat this position about five times. If you want to stretch even farther, while holding your ankles with your hands, place your forearms or elbows on the inside area of your thighs and push downward, as if you wanted your thighs to touch the floor. Maintain this position for twenty-five seconds (more if you can) and repeat it several times each day.

- Another similar exercise that also helps to increase flexibility in the pelvic area, and that helps your legs to open without difficulty at the time of delivery, consists of— beginning in the seated position described in the previous exercise—crossing the legs, one under the other, changing the cross-legged position every half a minute. Repeat five to ten times a day.

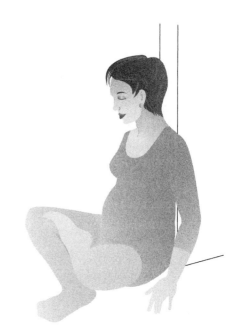

- A popular leg exercise (also for the pelvis and the back) is squatting. Hold on to something firm and try to squat down little by little. If this is difficult, begin by doing only half a squat—that is, place one leg in front of the other and squat down only on the leg you placed behind you, while the other remains with the sole of the foot on the floor. Rise slowly and change legs. When doing the

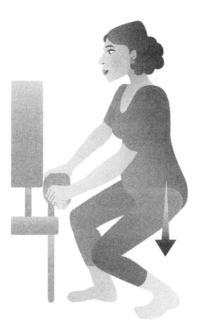

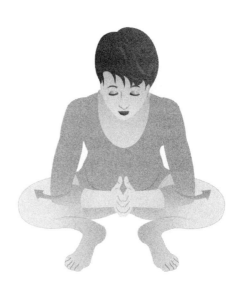

complete squat, remember to keep your back straight and to open your legs outward upon bending and lowering the body. If you are strong enough, do the squat without supporting yourself, open the legs and slightly point the ends of the feet outward; squat down and when you reach a comfortable position, stretch the bent legs outward, pushing them with your elbows from the inside of the thighs, at knee level (place your hands in a prayer position). The longer you stay there, the more benefit you will derive, as long as you don't tire yourself or experience any pain.

EXERCISES FOR THE ABDOMEN

- These are the only answer if you ever want to wear a bikini again after having your baby! Basically, they consist of raising your head up from the floor, or the bed,

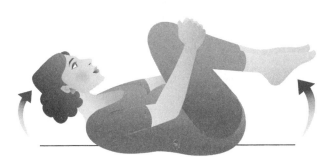

while you remain lying on your back with your knees bent. Also, in the same position, you can grab your knees with your hands and raise your head and shoulders, exhaling as you contract your abdominal muscles.

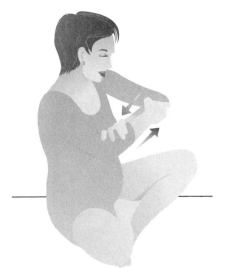

GENERAL EXERCISES
(Do every day, repeating each one ten times)

- Seated on the floor with legs crossed, grab each forearm with the opposite hand, and raise your elbows to shoulder level. Push each elbow with your hands until you feel the muscles below your breasts contract.

- Standing, with your back straight and holding on to something for support, raise one of your legs, straight, as high as is comfortably possible. Don't bend the other leg. Move the raised leg back and forth like a pendulum. Switch and do this with the other leg.

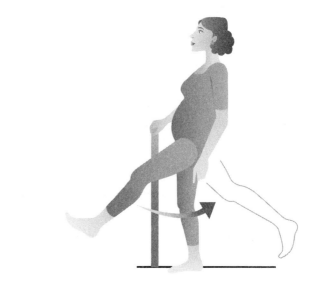

- Lying on your back on the floor, place your arms at your sides. Move your feet back in such a way as to raise your back up off the floor, with your buttocks in the air and your knees bent, legs slightly apart and the soles of your feet on the floor. Move the pelvis backward and forward, staying in each position for a few seconds. Breathe rhythmically.

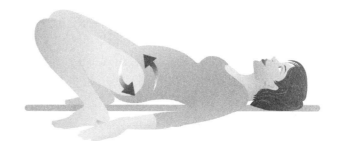

- Seated in a chair with your back straight and your hands on your thighs, move your head from side to side, as if you were trying to touch each ear to a shoulder (without raising the shoulder). Then, bring your head back, moving the neck from side to side; then move the neck in circles in both directions, and then make circles with your shoulders, forward and backward. All these movements should be done

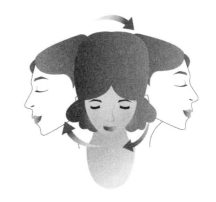

slowly, while maintaining rhythmic breathing, keeping the head in the different positions for a few seconds.

- Also seated, place your heels on the floor and push your toes downward while stretching only the big toe upward. Do this movement in reverse, big toe down and the others up.

- Seated, place your heels on the floor and move your feet in both directions, circling your heels outward and inward.

RELAXATION EXERCISES

Learning to relax both physically and mentally will not only help you endure any discomfort during the nine months, but will also help you be better prepared to face the birth of the baby. Selecting a comfortable position is the most important thing in doing these exercises. Many pregnant women achieve such a state of relaxation with these exercises that they sometimes fall asleep before finishing them!

Mental and physical relaxation go hand in hand, since your body and your mind form one whole. It's difficult to relax your muscles if you are not mentally relaxed; on the other hand, if you manage to relax your body you will have taken a huge step toward relaxing your mind. Some pregnant women find it easier to relax their bodies first, and others find it easier to relax their minds.

No matter which of these exercises you try, you will see how helpful they can be:

MENTAL RELAXATION

- Lie or sit in a quiet, restful place that is a comfortable temperature and dimly lit. If you like, you can listen to soft, relaxing music.

- Imagine that you have nothing to do in the next fifteen minutes, that you don't have to go anywhere, and that your whole world and all your interests are concentrated on the pleasant sensations you are about to experience.

- Close your eyes and focus your thoughts on the rhythm of your breathing, which should be slow and deep, but without effort.

- Try to eliminate all thoughts from your mind—this will help you imagine how the air slowly enters and exits your lungs.

- Try to think about pleasant things; beautiful landscapes you have visited or imagined, pleasant experiences (but not exciting ones). Some very relaxing images are the ocean, a peaceful creek, a sky with clouds, a valley seen from above, a waterfall, etc.

- If you are assaulted with a negative thought, superimpose an image of something pleasant over it. For example, as soon as you get a negative thought, imagine a huge bright blue sign in your mind that says "PEACE," or "LOVE," or "CHILD," or the name you plan to give your baby.
- Follow the rhythm of your breathing and concentrate on it. Mentally check all the areas in your body and assure yourself that there are no tense muscles. Do these exercises every other day for fifteen minutes at a time.

PHYSICAL RELAXATION

- Lie down or sit very comfortably where no one will bother you. Close your eyes and relax mentally, using the above techniques.
- Focus your mind on your right hand.
- Without moving from your position, tense the muscles of that hand, squeezing them slightly.
- Suddenly let go of those muscles and allow them to relax, maybe moving the hand slightly in order to release the tension you created before.
- Imagine that hand now being very, very heavy and warm. Imagine that hand is sinking slightly into the surface on which it is resting.
- Do the same thing with the forearm, the arm, the shoulder, the neck, the face, the foot, the leg, the inner thigh, the buttock, and the pelvis, and so forth until you have covered the entire right side of your body.
- Repeat this process with the left side of the body, always maintaining a calm, steady breathing rhythm.

LUCÍA MÉNDEZ

Actress (*Señora Tentación, Marielena, El extraño retorno de Diana Salazar, Tres veces Sofía, Golpe bajo*) and singer

Being pregnant is a very special sensation. Personally, I felt that the baby would be exactly the way my son, Pedro Antonio, is today. I knew, I don't know why, before they did the ultrasound, that it would be a boy and that his personality, from the start, would be strong. I felt that I was physically and morally sharing my spirit with my son.

I believed mine would be a natural vaginal delivery, but I never thought having a child would hurt so much, so I "chickened out" and asked for a cesarean. Naturally, I kept a diet and exercised throughout the pregnancy; that's why I only gained nine kilos (about twenty pounds) during the whole process, which helped me not to feel too heavy and to recover quickly.

Chapter 5

DISCOMFORTS
OF PREGNANCY

During pregnancy your body is experiencing many changes. These changes, which manifest in various ways, both physically and psychologically, sometimes produce a certain malaise or discomfort. Although it is common to experience some of the discomforts I will describe in the following pages, it is important that you share them with your doctor during your visits, or call him or her if they are severe. Since we're all different, these discomforts may vary from month to month and from one woman to another.

PHYSICAL DISCOMFORTS

GENERAL DISCOMFORT

Fatigue and sleepiness

Some of the first things you will notice are more common during the first months and toward the end of the pregnancy. In fact, it would be strange not to feel tired, since your body is actively at work—so much so that pregnancy has been compared with the effort it takes to climb a mountain. Your body is especially intensely occupied with the making of the placenta, the protective organ that will nurture the baby.

Try to get as much rest as possible in order to give your body the opportunity to recover. Naturally there is no need to overdo it; although you may find it odd, sometimes the more you rest, the wearier you feel. If this is your first baby, take advantage of the solitude and sleep now for all the time you will be unable to sleep once the baby is born! Go to bed earlier and, if you choose to, nap during the day. Take it easy.

Don't forget to exercise, as I recommended earlier. At least walk a few blocks a day. If you are extremely tired, you may be anemic. In other words, your red blood cell count could be low. In this event, your doctor can recommend treatment.

Dizziness and fainting

Some women get dizzy or faint. Some don't. These symptoms occur when there is a decrease in the blood flow to the brain, which temporarily decreases the amount of oxygen reaching the brain. It could happen because the uterus is using a lot more blood than normal and/or because the blood is taking longer to reach the brain—for instance, if you get up from a chair or rise out of bed very quickly to answer the phone.

It can also happen when you stand for long periods, especially in very crowded and warm places. For example, while you stand in line at the supermarket. Have you noticed that, in the films of the forties, you always knew when the woman was pregnant because she would faint? According to the experts, though, Hollywood screenwriters were not well informed. Weariness and dizziness are a surer sign of pregnancy than are fainting spells. If you feel dizzy or as though you might faint, sit down and place your head between your knees, or lie down with your feet up so they are at a higher level than your head. If you do faint, call your doctor that same day.

Dizziness or fainting could also be due to a low sugar level in the blood. That's why it is recommended not to let too many hours go by without eating (include snacks between meals). For example, always carry a small box of raisins, a piece of fruit, crackers, or bread to eat when you feel a little hungry.

Morning sickness

Morning sickness is the infamous nausea and vomiting that some pregnant women suffer, especially during the first three months. Even though it is known as morning sickness, it can happen at any time of day.

Nausea and vomiting are normal and happen to 50 percent of pregnant women. Morning sickness is believed to be caused by hormonal changes. Tiredness may contribute to more severe bouts of nausea.

Avoid eating too much too quickly, as a preventive measure, or at least to alleviate the problem. Choose foods with a high protein content and carbohydrates such as whole grain breads, lentils, beans, roasted or baked potatoes in their jackets, cheese, and milk. Avoid looking at, smelling, or tasting strong foods, perfumes, toothpaste, or anything that makes you nauseated.

The best thing to do when it happens is to relax and believe that the symptoms will go away on their own, just as they came. Avoid taking medication, unless recommended by your doctor. Estimates show that only about 7 of every 2,000 pregnant women suffer such severe nausea as to warrant using medication.

MYTH: A SCARE MAY CAUSE IMMEDIATE LABOR

If this were true, the number of women renting horror movies during the final month of pregnancy would escalate tremendously. In fact, stores would offer a section of "videos to induce labor within twenty-four hours."

Contractions

Some women feel contractions, known as Braxton Hicks contractions, toward the beginning of the pregnancy (in the fourth month). However, most feel them at seven or eight months. They are caused by the uterine muscles, which are "practicing" for the moment when they must go into action.

Contractions feel like a uterine spasm that is not necessarily painful, but can be uncomfortable. They usually last thirty seconds, although they can go for as long as two minutes. As your pregnancy reaches term, contractions increase in frequency and sometimes can be painful.

Changing position, either walking or lying down, could ease the discomfort. If the contractions are very frequent (let us say more than four per hour) and if they are accompanied by back or pelvic and stomach pain, call your doctor because you could be going into premature labor.

PAIN

Headaches

Headaches are more frequent during the first three months, but there are women who suffer from them throughout the pregnancy. There are many causes, including nasal congestion, fatigue, caffeine withdrawal, and anxiety. Headaches, though uncomfortable, are normal, unless you realize the pain is sharp, severe, and/or affects your vision. These more severe headaches, especially toward the end of the pregnancy, could indicate preeclampsia. Alert your doctor if you are having severe headaches.

To fight or alleviate the problem, try to rest. Work on your relaxation exercises. Try putting hot, damp compresses on your eyes and forehead. And ask your doctor if you may take a small dosage of acetaminophen (Tylenol, Datril, etc.).

Back pain

Generally backaches occur in the middle or toward the end of the pregnancy. The shape and balance of your body shift little by little as the months go by and you change the way you stand and sit. These new positions of your bones and muscles, and of your body in general, can cause muscular tension.

Around the eighth month, the baby may press against your spine, causing pain or "stabs" in the lower part of your back. These pains can radiate down into one or both legs and reach one or both feet.

Some recommendations to prevent or alleviate backache are as follows:

- Try, as much as possible, to maintain good posture (see the previous chapter for some advice on exercises for the posture). In spite of the fact that the increase in the size of the abdomen may make you prone to throwing your head and shoulders back, always attempt to keep a straight spine, perpendicular to the ground; this effort may be helped if you contract the muscles of your buttocks and abdomen.
- When sitting, always try to keep your feet up and your spine straight; sit up straight and keep your back erect (it might be useful to place a little pillow in the small of your back).
- Avoid any exertion. For example, do not bend at the waist to pick something up; you should bend your knees in order to get closer to the floor.
- Choose chairs with straight backs, and place a pillow in the small of your back if the chair where you like to sit tends to "sink."

- Lie on your back on firm mattresses when you rest, and give yourself gentle massages.
- To alleviate an ache in the upper back, rotate your head and shoulders (see Chapter 4, The Benefits of Exercise).
- And, possibly the most important advice: Avoid excessive weight gain.

Abdominal pain

From mid-pregnancy to term, you may experience pain on the sides of the pelvis. What is happening is that the muscles and ligaments of your body that support the uterus are being stretched. You will feel the pain particularly when you get out of bed or up from a chair or when you cough.

As long as the pain is slight, not constant, and not accompanied by vaginal discharge, fever, bleeding, or other symptoms, there is no need for concern. However, pain in the lower abdomen could mean a bladder infection, for instance. It's important to mention any symptom to your doctor. If you notice abdominal pain, change position, try sleeping on your side or try using a hot water bottle wrapped in a towel. If it is severe and persists, notify your doctor.

Aching bones and joints

During pregnancy your joints become less solid. Therefore, it's normal that your knees may suddenly buckle or your ankles twist. As the pregnancy advances, your chest cavity also expands and you could experience sudden and fleeting jabs to your ribs. This is the uterus pressing against your rib cage. For these reasons, wearing low-heeled shoes during pregnancy, walking calmly, and watching where you step are recommended. If you feel pain in your ribs, try to stretch out—either lying, standing, or sitting. Keeping good posture also means giving the baby you are carrying more room in your abdomen.

EYESIGHT

It is possible that you may experience vision problems or, more commonly, that existing problems (such as myopia) worsen. Sometimes pregnant women experience intolerance to the use of contact lenses; in these cases ophthalmologists recommend the use of glasses at least temporarily.

THE MOUTH

Tooth decay

If you have cavities, it is important to have them filled. Local anesthesia will not affect the baby, and a tooth infection would be worse. Avoid X-rays during pregnancy, but make sure to go for a dental exam and cleaning before and/or during pregnancy.

Due to the high concentration of hormones during pregnancy, the gums are more prone to swelling and bleeding. The best way to prevent dental problems is to brush your teeth at least twice a day.

Excessive saliva

Excessive salivation is another common symptom in pregnancy. Although the cause is unknown, it is basically a harmless discomfort that usually disappears after the first three months. It seems to be more common in pregnant women who also suffer from morning sickness.

THE SKIN

Rashes

Sometimes rashes can appear during pregnancy, especially on covered areas where sweating occurs. Sometimes they can cause itching. Keep those areas dry with talcum powder or cornstarch (Maizena), or use calamine lotion.

Blotches and discoloration

Few women escape some skin changes during pregnancy. These are caused by the high level of hormones in the body. Frequently these stains disappear after giving birth. For example, some women notice blotches on the nose, cheeks, or forehead, which may be somewhat noticeable and may cover an area similar to the "mask on a raccoon." Very often, there is a darkening of the nipples and the surrounding skin, or of the skin on the inside of the thighs; a line may also appear from the navel down to the pubic area.

Avoid long exposures to the sun as this increases the intensity of the blotches (aside from the fact that excessive exposure to the sun's rays is not recommended for anybody). If you do sunbathe, use a sunblock with a sun protection factor of at least 15 (15 SPF), and wear a hat.

Stretch marks

Stretch marks—those long pink or reddish marks that appear on the skin of breasts, abdomen, and hips and are caused by the stretching of the skin—are the horror of women who like the beach or the swimming pool. Unfortunately, they occur in 90 percent of pregnant women.

Those women who inherited skin with more elasticity than most are lucky, for they can have many children and never have a single stretch mark on their bodies. But they are the exceptions.

Generally speaking, there is no cream, lotion, or oil—no matter how expensive it is— that prevents 100 percent the appearance of stretch marks, although massage with cocoa butter may help. This does not mean that creams are not good in order to keep the skin lubricated. After delivery, stretch marks become fine, pale-colored lines that are less visible.

It's also important to avoid excessive weight gain.

MYTH: APPLYING OIL ON THE ABDOMEN TWICE A DAY PREVENTS STRETCH MARKS (THE LINES CAUSED BY SKIN STRETCHING)

Although it is true that applying cream or oil daily may help maintain healthier skin and diminish the possibility of developing stretch marks, there are other contributing factors. One example is the speed with which weight is gained— women who gain a lot of weight or gain weight quickly are more likely to develop stretch marks. A genetic factor involving elasticity of the skin is also important.

Acne

Due to the hormones in your body, your skin will secrete more oils during these months. That is the reason why many mothers appear "radiant," especially those with dry skin who benefit from these changes. However, women with oily skin may develop acne, of the type that appears days before a menstrual period. The good news is, the skin goes back to normal after delivery.

OTHER PROBLEMS

Common symptoms, considered normal and not requiring treatment since they disappear after delivery, include:

- Itching of the palms and soles of the feet, with or without reddening of the skin
- Fragile nails with a tendency to tear
- Bluish blotches on the legs when you feel cold

THE DIGESTIVE SYSTEM

Heartburn, acidity in the stomach, or indigestion

You may notice them from mid-pregnancy through term. As the uterus grows, it pushes the stomach upward, which makes the stomach acids rise, too. In addition, during the pregnancy the digestive system usually slows down. To prevent or alleviate these problems, the following is recommended:

- Eat small quantities of nutritious foods several times a day, instead of three large meals.
- Avoid excessive spices and fried foods.
- Do not smoke (for this and many other reasons).
- Relax and sleep with a pillow that will hold your head up six inches.
- Generally avoid wearing tight clothing, especially around the waist.
- Avoid lying down or exercising right after eating.
- Try to avoid baking soda; it contains a large amount of salt and this will cause you to retain fluids.
- Consult with your doctor to determine whether medication is necessary.

Gas

Precisely because the intestines are lazier, it is more difficult to eliminate the air that you swallow or that is produced by the digestion of certain foods such as beans, onions, and fried foods. Many mothers are concerned that the pressure of their uncomfortable and swollen stomach will bother the baby. Relax . . . the only one who is uncomfortable is you. The baby is comfortable and happy, protected by the fluid that surrounds it, and totally unaware of the sacrifices you are making on his or her behalf. The recommendations to diminish gas include the following:

- Do not eat too much at each meal.
- Chew your food well and avoid swallowing foods in large chunks.
- Eat slowly and avoid foods that can produce gas, including fried foods, beans, lentils, chick peas, cauliflower, and broccoli, among others.

Constipation

Constipation is more common after the midway point of the pregnancy. On the one hand, as your uterus grows, it takes up space normally belonging to the digestive system. On the other hand, the hormones make your bowel movements slower.

This does not mean you should sit back and suffer. There are several things you can do:

- Eat a lot of fiber (raw fresh fruits and vegetables, with their skins; whole grain cereals; rye bread; legumes; dried fruits such as prunes and dehydrated peaches).
- Drink large quantities of liquids, especially water and fruit and vegetable juices. Prune juice is especially effective. An old home remedy is to take a teaspoonful of olive oil before meals, or (according to some of my patients) to prepare an elder plant infusion. However, there is no scientific study to corroborate the latter, so I don't recommend it.
- Exercise daily. For example, take a walk.
- Avoid taking laxatives; they irritate the intestines.

Hemorrhoids

Another of the discomforts caused by the growing uterus and the increase in the blood flow toward the vagina and the rectum is hemorrhoids. Constipation doesn't help, as the effort required in moving the bowels increases the pressure and contributes to a weakening of the anal blood vessels. Hemorrhoids are varicose veins in the area of the anus and rectum. Do not ignore this problem.

The first thing to avoid is constipation (see the suggestions above). To treat hemorrhoids, use cotton with a little warm water or running water and soap to clean the area after you have had a bowel movement. A special ointment prescribed by your doctor, or ice cubes wrapped in a handkerchief and applied to the area will offer temporary relief. Practice the Kegel exercises, which consist of contracting the muscles in that area as if you were interrupting a flow of urine, holding for ten to thirty seconds, then releasing. Repeat several times. Do this exercise fifty times a day. It will help strengthen the vaginal and anal muscles.

Cravings and rejecting certain foods

Traditionally, it has been said that if a mother does not satisfy her sudden craving for a particular food, her child will be born with a birthmark in the shape of the food she craved and didn't eat. Now we know that none of this is true and that the marks some children have at birth are from other causes.

What is true is that pregnant women tend to crave certain foods and reject others. The real cause is unknown. Craving and rejecting might be due to hormonal changes, a nutritional deficiency the body tries to fulfill, or an emotional need to be pampered during a time of great insecurity, which a pregnancy surely can be. The real cause remains a mystery. I have had couples in which the *father* claims to have had cravings before his wife knew she was pregnant. According to what they tell me, the men's cravings began precisely at the time when conception supposedly occurred and disappeared after the delivery.

Whatever the cause, all the experts agree that the best "treatment" for cravings is to satisfy them whenever possible and, for food that is rejected, not to force the future mother to eat what she doesn't want.

THE RESPIRATORY TRACT

Shortness of breath

While the baby is in the upper part of the uterus—in other words, mid-pregnancy to the middle of the ninth month—you will notice that, no matter how hard you breathe, you will always feel you lack air. This happens because the baby is squeezing your lungs and exerting pressure on the diaphragm. This does not mean that you or your baby is not getting enough oxygen.

If you feel you are lacking air, do the following exercise: Raise your arms above your head and stretch upward; breathe slowly and deeply, hold your breath about four seconds, then slowly release the air. Do things calmly and take your time. It is better to arrive late . . . than out of breath.

If you notice a sudden or progressive difficulty in breathing, if you notice your lips are blue, or if you have a pain in your chest, go to the emergency room immediately.

Asthma

If you are asthmatic and are under medical supervision, you need not be too concerned about your pregnancy. However, even though asthma has a minimal effect on a pregnancy, the pregnancy can affect an asthmatic mother. Depending on your individual case, your asthma may improve, worsen, or remain the same. In any event, it is important that you avoid the factors that you know cause an asthma attack (e.g., dust, mildew, cats or dogs, perfumes, cigarette smoke, etc.). Do not smoke under *any* circumstances. Try to avoid catching any colds or flus. Ask your doctor if you should be vaccinated against influenza. If you suffer an asthma attack, use your inhaler immediately. In this event, the lack of oxygen resulting from an asthma attack is more dangerous than using your medication.

THE CIRCULATORY SYSTEM

Nosebleeds and nasal congestion

Just as in many other parts of the body, the increased flow of blood fills the mucous membranes of the nose in such a way that they may become swollen. This symptom could worsen and not disappear until the baby is born. If you live in a very cold climate, with dry, hot air from heaters in winter, the discomfort could increase. Using a dab of Vaseline on the inside of the nasal passages daily, before going to bed, could help prevent the dryness. Avoid blowing your nose too hard. If a nosebleed starts, stop the hemorrhage by squeezing your nose for a few minutes. Applying a handkerchief soaked with ice water may also help.

Varicose veins

Just like the veins of the rectum, the walls of the veins in the legs tend to relax and give way to the torrent of blood flowing through them. Therefore, they begin to bulge and to become visible through the skin. Toward the end of the pregnancy they may become more swollen. If there is a family history of varicose veins, or if you are overweight, you will be more prone to developing varicose veins. Recommendations for preventing them follow:

- Avoid standing for extended periods, especially if you are not moving.
- Avoid crossing your legs when sitting.
- Avoid remaining seated in the same position for extended periods.
- Avoid eating too much salt, which induces your body to retain fluids.
- Use support hose, available in maternity stores, which help the blood flow back from the legs against gravity.
- Exercise daily (for example, walk thirty or more minutes), which will stimulate circulation.
- Whenever you sit or lie down, keep your legs up.

High blood pressure

Although very few women experience high blood pressure during pregnancy, it does tend to go up around the seventh month. Often, too, you become nervous before seeing the doctor and your pressure reads somewhat high. If you suffered from high blood pressure before becoming pregnant, you must talk to your doctor to make sure the medication you are taking is not harming the baby. Most important, if you suffer from high blood pressure and are controlling it with medication, do not discontinue it without consulting your doctor. This could cause you and the baby problems.

Now, if you suddenly gain a lot of weight (more than three pounds in a week after the sixth month) and your hands and face become swollen, notify your doctor; this could be a symptom of preeclampsia, a serious condition that endangers the mother's life (see Chapter 3, preeclampsia and toxemia).

THE EXTREMITIES
Cramps

Leg cramps are frequent, especially during the final three months of the pregnancy. They could be due to the changes in the metabolism of calcium, or changes in the circulation within the muscles. If you get a cramp in your calf, consider these suggestions:

- Stretch the leg forward with the heel. Tell the person next to you to apply pressure on your knee with one hand and with the other to push against the sole of your foot.
- You may also rub and warm the leg to reactivate circulation.
- Do not lie on your back, because the weight of the uterus increases the pressure on the blood vessels that control the circulation in the leg.

Swelling

Also known as edema, the swelling of legs, feet, and hands is caused by fluid retention, something absolutely normal, which is due, partly, to sluggish circulation. The problem increases if you wear tight clothing around your ankles and feet.

Avoid excessive intake of salt, because that will only increase fluid retention. Put your legs up when sitting, don't stand for a long time, and wear loose clothing.

THE VAGINA

Normally during the pregnancy there is a small amount of secretion or vaginal discharge that is not uncomfortable. Due to the hormonal level, the normal acidity of the vagina becomes more alkaline and causes the woman to be more prone to certain vaginal infections caused by fungus. To diminish the risk of developing a fungal infection, wear loose clothing that allows the flow of air between the legs (this is no time for wearing tight pants!), wear cotton underwear, and take frequent warm baths. Avoid vaginal douches completely.

If the discharge smells strongly or causes pain or itching, call your doctor. Nonprescription creams may be recommended (not to be used, however, without your doctor's authorization). To reduce the itching, eat yogurt (some women even apply yogurt to the outside of the vagina).

If you notice bleeding, whether severe or just spotting, call your doctor that same day.

THE URINE

Frequent urination and infections

You will soon notice that you must urinate more frequently than before. This will happen in the initial stages of the pregnancy because the growing uterus is applying pressure to your bladder. Also, toward term, it increases because the baby descends, applying even more pressure.

Do not stop drinking water to diminish the number of times you visit the bathroom. On the contrary, drink more water and, if you like, drink cranberry juice, which helps prevent the bladder infections (cystitis) so common during pregnancy. The most common symptom of bladder infection is a burning sensation when you urinate. Treatment requires an antibiotic that your doctor will prescribe. To reduce the possibilities of infection, try these suggestions:

- Wipe from front to back after you finish urinating.
- Wear cotton underwear so that your skin breathes and humidity is avoided.
- Empty your bladder completely each time you go to the bathroom.

Sugar in the urine

As long as the sugar in the blood remains normal, the presence of sugar in the urine is of no consequence. If sugar is found in the urine, however, the level of sugar in the blood should be checked. It could be a sign of diabetes, which is highly prevalent in Latinas (see Chapter 3).

MENTAL HEALTH

DEPRESSION AND IRRITABILITY

Most women confuse depression with the normal symptoms of irritability and mood swings directly associated with all pregnancies. If you have always had mood swings prior to your period, and if, in general, you are a susceptible individual, the first three months of your pregnancy will be like suffering a continuous and increased period of PMS (pre-menstrual syndrome). If to that we add the physical symptoms of pregnancy, you will have every right to feel occasionally upset or irritable.

Now, if your upset persists, if you are not happy with your pregnancy, or if you are insecure, you could be in danger of falling into a depression. Ask yourself the following questions:

- Is there a history of depression in your family?
- Are there financial problems in the home?
- Do you have a high-risk pregnancy?
- Are you lacking support either from the baby's father or your family?
- Are you afraid you and/or the baby are not healthy?

If you answer yes to one or more of these questions, and in addition, you don't eat or sleep well, cannot concentrate, have lost interest in everything, or cry frequently, it is important that you talk to your doctor. Perhaps he or she may refer you to a psychologist or psychiatrist. In spite of these discomforts, this is a time of happiness, not a time for feeling blue.

INSOMNIA

In addition to the physical discomforts—cramps, aches, a baby that kicks, etc.—causing an inability to sleep, there are psychological aspects. You will lie awake and ask yourself what your life will be like with the new baby, and think about your financial situation, work concerns, and a thousand other things that make sleeping impossible. Or, perhaps your body is unconsciously preparing you for the lack of sleep you will experience for the first few months of your baby's life at home. Insomnia could also be a response to the great excitement you feel.

To diminish the possibility of insomnia: Try to eat lightly at night, exercise regularly, and avoid caffeine.

If you cannot sleep, leave the bedroom and read, relax, and wait until you feel sleepy. Do not take sleeping pills. Perhaps a cup of chamomile or linden tea will help or, at least, will ease your mind.

The best sleeping position during pregnancy is on your side, preferably the left, with one leg crossed over the other and a pillow between your knees. This position allows better blood circulation within the placenta and reduces the buildup of fluid in the legs, decreasing swelling.

LOSS OF MEMORY

If you leave your keys inside the car, your checkbook on the counter at the store, the milk out of the fridge, your jacket at the doctor's office . . . don't worry. No, you are not losing your mind! As with so many other things about your pregnancy, blame the hormones. The excitement and concern about the pregnancy can also be contributing factors. Be practical, and make a memory list: Write down everything important that you must do, especially things like locking the door. Remember, this is temporary and you are not the only one it's happening to.

DREAMS

With pregnancy, you will probably enter a private world of fantasy through your dreams. This is the way in which your subconscious releases the anxiety your mind accumulates during the day—through pleasant dreams or nightmares.

Many of the dreams experienced by pregnant women include things such as forgetting to feed the baby, being attacked by someone, leaving the baby behind, losing the baby, being trapped somewhere, being abandoned by their husbands because they look ugly, finding their husbands with lovers, or having a baby that is born deformed or sick. Don't allow any of this to frighten you, and remember . . . *dreams are only dreams.* Don't take them out on those around you as if they were real.

CRAVINGS

See earlier in this chapter, in the digestive system.

CHANGES IN YOUR BODY

THE BREASTS
Changes in size

As the pregnancy advances, your breasts will grow. The mammary glands, those that will produce the milk, will be filling with fluid. Also, fat deposits will increase in the body, including in the breasts. At this time, blue veins will appear, announcing an increase in the blood supply. Your breasts will be very sensitive and you will feel they are taut, hard, and heavy. They may even hurt.

Wearing a bra that supports without crushing will help. Choose cotton bras so that your skin breathes well, and increase the bra size as necessary.

Appearance of colostrum

After the fifth month your breasts may begin to produce colostrum at any time. This is a yellowish or transparent liquid, which is what will feed your baby. It is also normal if it doesn't appear until the final stages of pregnancy. The only discomfort is that you could be out when suddenly your blouse or dress becomes wet.

Clean your nipples with warm water and do not use soap that will irritate them. Place gauze or absorbent cotton over the nipples inside the bra. Pads specially designed for this purpose are available in pharmacies or maternity shops.

Inverted nipples

Having inverted nipples does not mean you will be unable to feed your baby when the time comes. Your doctor will recommend you use a special pump sold in maternity shops if he or she believes it is necessary.

THE ABDOMEN

If you have an enviable, tiny waist, say good-bye to it—temporarily—as this is the first thing to disappear during pregnancy. This change can be a consequence of the growth of the uterus, or can be caused by the distention of the intestines, which is very common in the initial stages. Or it could simply mean you are gaining weight. Remember that, by the second month, you should have gained about three pounds.

As the baby grows, it must settle and make proper use of the space within your uterus. During the seventh month, if the baby is placed as it should be—head down—your abdomen will be bulging upward. Later it will start going down.

If the size of your stomach bothers your sleep, try to rest on your side, bending your bottom leg inward (rest it against your stomach) and stretching out the upper leg. This position is recommended only for sleeping. For resting during the day, try to do so on your back and with your feet higher than the level of your body.

SPECIAL PROBLEMS

ANEMIA

Anemia is the result of a decrease in the red blood cell count, frequently due to a lack of iron (although there are other causes). During pregnancy the volume of blood increases and, with it, the amount of iron the body requires. Many women do not consume sufficient iron to cover this increased need, and therefore can present symptoms of anemia:

- Paleness
- Extreme fatigue
- Palpitations
- Weakness
- Fainting spells

Women who are expecting twins, who have had one baby after another in close succession, or who vomit frequently are more susceptible to developing anemia.

Depending on your case, your doctor may prescribe iron supplements (pills). However, the best way of taking iron is straight from foods rich in iron such as dry fruit, duck, beef, liver, oysters, sardines, squash, artichokes, and spinach. A blood sample can tell your doctor whether you are suffering from anemia.

ALLERGIES

To many women who suffer from allergies, pregnancy can increase the condition. Symptoms can include sneezing, watery eyes, or a stuffy nose (which could be confused with the normal symptom of congestion due to pregnancy). Even though allergies complicate the mother-to-be's existence, they are not a serious problem.

Aside from consulting your allergist, try to avoid—now more than ever—things that you know give you allergies. For instance:

- Keep your house dust-free.
- Use air-conditioning to avoid pollen in the house.
- Do not use down pillows.
- Avoid foods you are allergic to.
- If your pet is to blame, send the dog or cat to live elsewhere for a time.

OVARIAN CYSTS

One out of ten pregnancies produces benign ovarian cysts that, nonetheless, must be monitored to ensure they are not growing. In fact, those cysts almost never create problems, unless they threaten to burst. In this last case, your doctor may suggest surgical removal.

COLDS

Although there is some flu medication that can be taken during pregnancy, don't take anything (even if sold over the counter) without first consulting your doctor. Other things which may help are:

- Try to get a lot of rest and eat well.
- Drink a lot of liquids.

- Gargle with salt water to relieve throat dryness.
- If you run a fever, take warm showers and don't cover yourself too much.

GERMAN MEASLES, MUMPS, AND CHICKEN POX

Even though most women either have had these diseases or have been vaccinated against them, there is a chance that you fall into neither of these groups. The only way the virus that causes one of these diseases can harm the baby during pregnancy is if you catch it during this time.

The symptoms for German measles include fever, swollen glands, and skin rashes, which generally appear three weeks after being in contact with someone with the disease. If you suspect this to be your case, consult your doctor immediately.

If you have never had or been vaccinated for mumps and think you may have been exposed, or if you develop the symptoms (fever, swollen glands, earache, or soreness when chewing), consult your doctor.

Chicken pox is indicated by the appearance of small hives, which go through different stages (red bumps with water inside, like blisters, and then a scab before disappearing).

In the event you develop any of these symptoms, notify your doctor immediately.

TOXOPLASMOSIS

The parasite that causes this infection is transmitted by raw meat (or meat not properly cooked), or by the feces of certain animals, such as cats. It is estimated that 1 to 2 of every 1,000 babies in the United States are born infected with this parasite, and that one-third of the population has been exposed and has developed antibodies against the disease. In these cases, there is no danger to the baby. There are certain precautions recommended to avoid infection in people who have not had it and to prevent problems for the infant during the pregnancy. (See Chapter 3, Environmental Factors.)

HEPATITIS

There are several types of hepatitis: The ones we are usually concerned with, because they can affect the baby during gestation, are hepatitis B and hepatitis C. They are transmitted through sexual intercourse or by coming in contact with the blood of someone who is carrying the virus. The infected person may not be aware of having it, as it often shows no symptoms. As for blood transfusions, the risk of infection in this manner is almost nil in the United States; at this time all donated blood is screened for the hepatitis B and C virus, among other things (see Chapter 3).

HEART DISEASE

Although many doctors prefer that their patients who suffer from serious coronary problems do not become pregnant (especially women in a higher age range), sometimes a woman with heart disease may inadvertently become pregnant and decide to have her baby.

If this is your case, the care you must take depends on the seriousness of your condition. In general, the idea is that you follow these points:

- Avoid emotional stress.
- If you smoke, quit. (You should have done this by now anyway.)
- Maintain a low-cholesterol and low-sodium (salt) diet.
- Avoid gaining excessive weight.
- Take the medication prescribed and approved by your doctor regularly.

PROBLEMS WITH THE PLACENTA

There are three types of problems that could occur with your placenta:

Placenta previa

This is when the placenta remains adhered to the lower part of the uterus, instead of the superior or lateral walls of the womb. This can cause problems at the time of delivery. Many cases must resort to a cesarean section.

Placenta accreta

This occurs when the placenta grows adhered within the walls of the uterus and does not separate from the uterine wall during the third phase of labor. This sometimes requires removing the uterus after delivery.

Abruptio placenta

In this case the placenta separates from the uterus prematurely. This occurs after twenty-eight weeks of pregnancy (if sooner, it is considered a miscarriage). Depending on the degree of separation, anything from complete rest to an emergency delivery may be recommended. In severe cases, it could be a very serious complication.

PREMATURE RUPTURE OF MEMBRANES (PROM)

The premature rupture of membranes, or the water breaking (as it is commonly called), refers to the breaking of the water before contractions begin. This may happen weeks or hours before delivery. If contractions begin at that moment, and it is your doctor's opinion that it is too early, you may be given something to arrest them. However, if your membranes break at thirty-seven weeks or later, and labor does not begin on its own, it is possible the doctor will induce contractions to begin labor at that time. In the absence of contractions, the doctor will make sure to rule out prolapse of the umbilical cord, a situation that would require correction. Compression of the cord could compromise the baby's circulation. In any case, monitoring the baby to prevent fetal distress is imperative, as is discarding or ruling out any possibility of infection.

SYMPTOMS OF MISCARRIAGE

Even though statistics show only 15 percent of pregnancies end in miscarriage (not an induced abortion), this can be a traumatic experience for the couple and one that all pregnant women should be prepared for. It is more common in women of forty or older, where the incidence increases by 30 to 45 percent.

Almost all miscarriages happen within the first three months of pregnancy, which is why they are often confused with a heavy menstrual cycle, accompanied by cramping pains and sometimes blood clots. The typical symptoms of a miscarriage are cramping pains in the lower abdomen and vaginal bleeding. Most miscarriages are complete. They may occasionally be partial and, in these cases, a D & C (dilation and curettage) is required to remove the remaining embryo and or placenta that was not expelled.

However, spotting during the first three months of pregnancy is very common and does not necessarily mean that a miscarriage will occur. Sometimes bleeding stops and the pregnancy reaches term normally. But, as the popular saying goes, it's better to be safe than sorry. Consult your doctor right away.

MARIBEL GUARDIA

Actress (*Prisionera de amor, Tú y yo, Adventuras en el tiempo*) and singer

The only special care I took during my pregnancy was simply to walk an hour on a daily basis, and eat a lot of fruit (so that the baby would be born clean), as well as using a lot of cream on my stomach and breasts. Unfortunately, among Latina women, knowing the sex of their baby through ultrasound is still not a custom, which is really silly! In my case, knowing that it was a boy (his name is Julián) helped me welcome him not only with the proper clothes but also with a bedroom decorated with the appropriate details.

The worst experience during my pregnancy was that, due to the inadequacies of my body, the delivery was by cesarean section. I was so afraid that, in order to give me courage, I began praying to the Virgin I had taken with me to the hospital. Because at that point, all you can do is put yourself in God's hands.

When they took my son out of my stomach and put him in my arms, I felt like God had come to Earth. I was aware of a very strong light that somehow announced that with him I would really experience the love of my spirit in such a profound way that it is going to make me become a better human being.

Among the care you must offer your baby is that if you are going to breast-feed, first use almond oil on your nipples, so they don't become irritated; read books that talk about how to care for your baby; go for walks frequently with him; put cream on his face; and cut his nails.

Chapter 6

PREPARING YOURSELF
FOR THE DELIVERY

HOW TO GET READY FOR "THE BIG EVENT"

For all the stories you might have heard, nobody can be absolutely sure how your labor and delivery will go—whether it will be painful, easy, or difficult. Giving birth is totally different for each woman, different for mothers and daughters in the same family, and even from one pregnancy to the next for the same woman.

However, you cannot let fear dominate you, because then it *will* be difficult. Experience shows that women who are well informed on what may happen the day of the delivery are best prepared and encounter the least number of problems.

There are certain steps you can take from the start so the logical fears are easier to confront.

- Find a doctor who gives you proper attention and who answers all your questions and doubts concerning your condition, even though you may sometimes think they are silly.
- Sign up for a prenatal course at your hospital.
- Read books and magazines on pregnancy and labor.

- Share your fears and expectations regarding the delivery with your partner, family, and friends.

- Don't be ashamed of fearing pain. That is natural. What is absurd is to think that you will not feel pain or, at least, some discomfort. In this sense, being prepared is the best way to confront it.

- Learn relaxation and breathing techniques that will help manage the pain during labor. Knowing how to manage pain is extremely important; however, don't believe this will protect you against all the discomforts of labor. In any labor and delivery the mother-to-be, no matter how prepared she is, is incapable of completely controlling her body. Part of the process includes certain unconscious or involuntary mechanisms. For example, you cannot determine the number of your contractions, but you can be prepared to face them, however many there are.

- Remember that the process of giving birth is very intense, from both a physical and an emotional point of view. And, in the same way you may lose control over your body, you may lose control over your emotions. But none of that is important: Do not worry if you suddenly scream or feel out of control. The medical personnel caring for you are there to help. Remember: After nine months of pregnancy you are not in the hospital to behave well, but to give birth. And, although you obviously want to cooperate as much as possible, your only job is to make everything right for you and your baby. Forget the rest.

- Ask your doctor about anesthesia. Although many women are capable of handling the pain without the need for an anesthetic, it is convenient (and comforting) to be informed that alternatives are available. These alternatives offer advantages and disadvantages (see Chapter 11).

- Visit the hospital's delivery rooms, where you will be giving birth, beforehand, so that you will be familiar with the place when the moment comes.

- And, finally, realize that, no matter how much you plan, a delivery can always present unexpected situations. No matter how much you practice breathing, it's possible that, at the last minute, the intensity of the pain will prompt you to request an anesthetic. Though you may have decided on a natural birthing process, it's possible that, when the moment comes, your doctor will be forced to perform a cesarean section. **But never lose sight that giving birth—no matter how difficult it may be, and even though you may not be in as much control as you would wish—is the** most extraordinary experience of your life. You have had the privilege of giving and receiving this most wonderful of gifts, the life of a human being . . . your son or daughter.

PLACE OF BIRTH AND NATIONALITY

Babies born while the mother is traveling between countries—by train, ship, or plane—have the right (according to international law) to carry the nationality of the carrier company on which the birth takes place as well as the nationality of the parents.

BIRTHING CLASSES

There was a time when all women gave birth at home, and deliveries were not considered a medical event. In the past, things were simpler . . . but also more dangerous, especially if there were complications. Fortunately, medicine intervened, in many cases, to save the lives of the mother and her baby. At the same time, in Europe, classes were developed to train the mother-to-be, and the baby's father, and to make her ready for her sublime moment.

OBJECTIVES AND BENEFITS
- Educating the parents so that they will be well informed before entering the delivery room
- Diminishing the anxiety and natural fear in most women, and helping them share thoughts with other pregnant women
- Preparing women for physical pain with breathing and relaxation methods
- Explaining to the mother-to-be what to expect at the onset of labor, and showing her the delivery room and how it functions
- Teaching her exercises to maintain the elasticity of her muscles
- Preparing the father so he may support his partner both physically and psychologically

EXERCISES

Aside from the exercises you can and must do alone at home, with your physician's approval (see Chapter 4), the prenatal classes will teach you stretching exercises as well as the different ways you could choose to give birth: whether squatting, sitting, or lying down. This is in conjunction with what you have discussed with your doctor. The exercises are important not only during the pregnancy to protect your body and your spine as they confront the growing weight they must deal with, but also at the moment of labor, when they are essential to keeping you relaxed and in good shape.

There are also yoga exercises, which emphasize breathing and yogi philosophy. Perhaps the most valuable exercises during these classes are those dealing with the lower pelvis, which will help the uterus have firmer support. There are also classes given in swimming pools, should you be interested. Swimming is also an excellent exercise for pregnant women.

THE LAMAZE METHOD

Lamaze is the most renowned of the methods that prepare pregnant women. It was popularized because it promised "a painless delivery." In truth, there is no delivery without some pain, but with Lamaze training well used, delivery can be rendered a lot easier and pain greatly controlled.

The Lamaze method is taught in group classes of approximately twelve women, with weekly practices starting in about the seventh month. In these classes, aside from offering information as to the development of the pregnancy and the delivery, exercises that strengthen and increase muscle flexibility are taught, as are relaxation and breathing exercises. Everything is geared so that the pregnant woman has more knowledge and control over her body when she reaches her big moment.

The breathing exercises are the foundation of the Lamaze method for it is, in fact, through controlled and forced breathing that the mother in labor will make her child come forth. The method is based in making the woman concentrate and breathe abdominally, deeply, and rhythmically at the moment of greatest stress during labor, to distract her attention from the pain and to have her mind respond automatically to the contractions as they take place.

However, it is not always easy to combine the painful uterine contraction with the breathing rhythm. Some of the Lamaze method advantages are

- Reduced awareness of pain
- Increased active participation by the woman in the process
- Stimulated participation by the father at the delivery as a "helper" during labor

THE LEBOYER METHOD

The objective of the Leboyer method is that the baby come into the world in a calm environment, with soft lighting and no noise, placing the child immediately over its mother's stomach for about five minutes with his umbilical cord intact. When it stops pulsating, it is cut, and the infant is held and bathed in warm water so it is not traumatized by the difference between the warm interior of the mother and the colder temperature of the outside world. It may be combined with the Lamaze method.

There are hospitals that refuse to turn down the lighting to the degree of softness this method demands, but there are many mothers who swear that, thanks to these suggestions, labor was far more pleasant. If you are interested in this, you may read a book called *Birth Without Violence* written by the creator of the method, Dr. Frederick Leboyer.

MYTH: IF THE MOTHER HAS BEEN SUDDENLY FRIGHTENED, THE BABY WILL HAVE A BIRTHMARK

One out of ten babies is born with a birthmark, either red or brown, which often appears on the face, the neck, the lower back, or the buttocks. Frequently, these birthmarks disappear during the first months of life. If every time the mother is suddenly frightened over the nine-month period of pregnancy was represented by a birthmark on her child, there would be pinto babies.

Also, within nine months, it is likely that all women have at least one fright; however, not all babies have birthmarks. This is part of the folklore that gets passed down but has no basis in science or medicine.

DELIVERY ALTERNATIVES

HOSPITAL DELIVERY

If you have a high-risk pregnancy (for example, a multiple pregnancy, or you have had complications in previous pregnancies), if you are over thirty-five, or if you have any sign or symptom suggestive of possible complications, it is not recommended that you consider delivery outside a hospital. Do not take any unnecessary risks. Doctors and traditional health centers are equipped for any eventuality.

The process at the clinic begins in the dilation room and continues in the delivery room (see Chapter 11). There is a small operating room next door should minor surgery be necessary, and, naturally there's a nursery with incubators and everything a newborn baby needs. There are hospitals where the mother's pleasant room suddenly becomes the delivery room when the moment arrives.

As for the doctors, you will suddenly see a whole lot of white laboratory coats, greens, and uniforms. This is the usual structure:

- Your obstetrician, or the doctor on call for him or her, is the head of the team and will be responsible for their coordination. He or she will be the one who receives the baby and performs any necessary surgery.
- The associate doctors will assist the chief doctor.
- Residents and new graduate doctors will be communicating with you, if you are in a university hospital or a teaching hospital.
- Depending on your case, a certified midwife or a specialized nurse may be helping you with moral support and guiding your breathing during contractions. According to the training and enthusiasm of the father, sometimes he is the one who plays this role.

This structure is common in larger hospital centers. In some smaller hospitals there are fewer personnel. The important thing is that you have your obstetrician with you, and if necessary, an anesthesiologist.

HOME DELIVERY

Many women, especially in recent years, are choosing to give birth at home, considering it a warmer and friendlier approach. Naturally, this decision has its advantages: You may feel more relaxed in your own environment; you don't need to go anywhere after giving birth; if you so wish, family members can participate; and the same midwife who has followed your pregnancy will be at your side to help you. The disadvantages: If for any reason, there is a complication during labor or delivery or if you decide that you want to be anesthetized, no qualified personnel with proper equipment will be available to act immediately.

The decision to deliver at home with a midwife must include confirmation that, within the realm of foreseeable possibilities, you will not require a cesarean section or the monitoring of the baby to avoid fetal distress, things that could only be accomplished at a hospital.

Even when everything seems to be going perfectly, you must be prepared to be taken to a hospital in the event of an emergency. Another consideration in the case of deliveries not within a hospital is that, often, you are responsible for all the expenses; most medical insurance plans do not cover home delivery. Insurance companies believe that, although on the surface the cost of home delivery seems much less, the risk of complications under these circumstances is greater.

> Only 7 percent of pregnancies come from women thirty-five and over at the time of delivery.

THE BABY'S PRESENCE

On every visit, your doctor will inform you how your baby is doing. Do not hesitate to ask questions if you have any doubts or concerns. The following are natural signs and routine examinations that will help reassure you the development of the baby is fine:

FETAL HEARTBEAT

At seventeen weeks, with the use of a stethoscope, you will be able to hear your baby's heartbeat. However, you should not worry if you don't hear it until much later. For example, if your abdomen has a thick layer of fatty tissue, the heartbeat will not be heard early on. In these cases, or if there is any doubt as to the baby's development, the doctor can perform an ultrasound test.

FETAL MOVEMENT

One of the greatest joys during pregnancy is when the expectant mother feels her baby move. That's why many mothers worry too much when this doesn't happen right away. Do not be concerned. Generally the baby's movements aren't felt until the fourteenth week, and many others don't feel them until the twenty-second week. A traditional (and not very scientific) way of knowing whether everything is fine with your baby is to count the times it moves; this system works only after the twenty-eighth week. The idea is to count how many times the baby moves in half a day (approximately twelve hours). Ten times or more seems to be the standard. If the baby moves a lot, it may be a soccer player! (This is not necessarily true, but many fathers would be delighted if it were, wouldn't they?) If the baby moves fewer than ten times within twelve hours after the twenty-eighth week, do not be concerned; however, if it does not move at all within that period, call your doctor.

Many women describe those first movements as an undulation or tickling in the stomach. As the baby grows, it starts to kick, and those are movements you will notice immediately. Some babies even wake their mothers in the middle of the night with the power of their kicks!

Do not worry if suddenly you don't feel your baby move. This doesn't mean it isn't moving, only that it is doing so more gently. Many babies are lulled during the day by their mother's coming and going, and they wake up at night.

FETAL HICCUPS

Many mothers feel gentle, regular spasms in their abdomens. This is not the baby kicking, but—believe it or not——the infant having an attack of hiccups. Especially during the final months. Some fetuses get hiccups on a daily basis. But don't be upset: Nothing bad will happen to a baby with hiccups. Unlike adults, they can overcome these attacks without a care. What's more, enjoy it and take it as a sign of your baby's good health.

HOW THE BABY ARRIVES

Around the eighth month, both mothers and their doctors must begin observing the baby's position. Most fetuses place themselves head down between thirty-two and thirty-six weeks, but some keep you guessing to the very end. If the baby is sitting, the doctor may try to change its position from the outside, with his or her own hands.

One of the amusements mothers-to-be engage in is trying to guess, according to the movements they feel, what position the baby is in: Are these the shoulders? the head? the feet? In fact, there is no way of being 100 percent sure of the position the baby will assume at the time labor begins. The weekly examination with your obstetrician during the last month of pregnancy is extremely important.

CLOTHING FOR MOTHER AND BABY

MATERNITY CLOTHES

Being pregnant does not mean that you must dress more soberly, or as if you were ill. Simply adapt your usual way of dressing to your new figure. For many pregnant women, this is a time to pamper themselves and buy new clothes, but that does not mean your whole wardrobe must be changed.

Having items that can be mixed and matched with many others is ideal. For instance, a favorite article of clothing of modern mothers is stretch pants, which can be worn under different jackets, blouses, and/or dresses to create new ensembles that look different every time.

Generally the following are recommended:

- Wear comfortable clothing that isn't tight on you, and avoid tight elastics. Avoid clothes that are tight around the waist or that decrease the blood flow in the legs. Remember that, as your breasts grow over the months (as will your tummy!), you will need dresses with a lot of room under the arms, at the height of the chest and the waist.
- Wear cotton underwear so your skin breathes well. Generally look for light and fresh cotton items or natural-fiber clothes (during the pregnancy you will be warmer than normal). However, if you feel cold or it is wintertime, do dress warmly with layers that you can remove if necessary.
- Wear a good bra, not simply a large one. It must fit snugly without being tight, should have wide straps (so that they don't leave marks on your shoulders), and should be made from natural fibers that won't cause itching.
- Ask your doctor about a maternity girdle for back support.
- Do not buy a lot of pants; some women find them uncomfortable during the last weeks of the pregnancy.

- Borrow clothes from friends who have already had babies.
- Use the clothes you wore before the pregnancy if they are wide, or make minimal alterations to them, right up to the fifth or sixth month of pregnancy. However, for many women, part of their own psychological well-being during this period is in the ability to wear "special maternity clothes."
- Remember that, if you have gained a lot of weight, materials with vertical lines and darker colors tend to help give you a slimmer figure.
- Don't wear clothing that isn't comfortable. Some women, during the first months of pregnancy, insist on wearing dresses than no longer fit—because they like them a lot—and they struggle until they manage to close them. Usually around the waist is the first place they will feel tight. Squeezing into too-small clothes is unhealthy; you won't feel comfortable, and you won't look good. . . . And you may even ruin the dress!
- Wear dresses that button down the front. They will also be very useful for breast-feeding after the birth.
- Have at least two bras that clasp in front, if you plan to breast-feed your baby. However, do not buy them until the final weeks of pregnancy as your breasts will continue growing and you will want to get the correct size.
- Discard shoes with very high heels. Your shoes should have low heels and be very comfortable, although they need not be completely flat. You will notice that lower heels are more comfortable. And, after the sixth month, forget tennis or jogging shoes that have laces and need to be tied up. Your stomach will probably not allow you to bend over!

BABY CLOTHES
- Diapers. Some experts advise the use of cotton diapers for the first few months of the baby's life. Cotton is softer than disposable diapers and allows you to know more quickly when your baby needs to be changed. Naturally, the throwaway is much more convenient for the mother, and more absorbent. The cost could influence your decision. Some people alternate between the two. Estimates indicate that using disposable diapers requires about six dozen a week. If you are using cloth diapers, you may want to cover them with a pair of rubber pants.
- Undershirts (five or six), sweaters (two or three), pajamas or sleepers (six or eight of the one-piece outfits—stretch suits—that unbutton down the front and along the

insides of both legs and allow easy changing of diapers), nightgowns (two or three), soft boots or socks (two to four), a woolly cap for winter or a light one for summer, bibs (two to four).

- Coverlets (two to four) to use either when going out or at home.
- Clothes should be made of nonflammable materials, as they are safer.

The baby's clothes should be washed separately from the adult clothes in the home and should never be washed with normal detergents. Use water and a liquid soap that doesn't have strong chemicals. Do not use bleach. All the clothes that come into direct contact with the baby's skin must be extremely soft, should not have buttons or rough stitching, and, if possible, should be made of natural fibers.

OTHER ARTICLES FOR THE BABY

You may spend as much money as you like on your baby, but the following are the first articles you should buy (starting the first months after birth), because they are basic necessities as soon as the baby arrives:

- An infant safety seat for the car. Some hospitals will not allow taking the baby home without an infant seat.
- Pacifiers (optional, not all parents like to use them, although many use them in the case of babies who cry a lot even after being fed).
- At least one baby bottle with which to give your baby water and, perhaps, a pump to extract milk with, should you decide to breast-feed. Pumps can be rented as well.
- Baby bottles with nipples, with which to feed your new child, should you not choose to breast-feed. Estimates show that four 4-ounce bottles and approximately ten 8-ounce bottles with newborn baby nipples is ideal. You will also need a sterilizer, if your doctor recommends one, and the necessary instruments with which to prepare your baby's formula. Your doctor will recommend the type of formula. You will probably want to buy enough formula to last one or two weeks at least.
- A crib with a firm mattress, plastic covered, and bedding (at least two changes) appropriate to the season. Select, above all, a soft and warm blanket. You don't need to buy pillows right away as, at least for the first few months after birth, they are not

recommended. Avoiding them at this time not only reduces the risk of suffocation, but also keeps the spine straight.

- Two to four very soft towels to dry your baby with, and two to four small towels (face towels) to wash it with.
- A portable bathtub.
- A thermometer to measure the temperature of the bathwater.
- Several bandages for the umbilical cord area, so that you can change them whenever it feels damp. Your doctor will instruct you on how to do this.
- A table for diaper changing.
- Grooming articles: comb and brush for the baby; sponge; very gentle liquid soap; cream and ointment for diaper rash (ask your doctor which he or she recommends); damp towels with which to wipe the baby when changing diapers; talcum powder or cornstarch; oil and/or Vaseline for the skin; cotton balls, preferably sterilized; six to eight safety pins (if using cloth diapers); and a round-tipped pair of scissors with which to trim the nails.
- A thermometer for the baby, and a small bottle of liquid acetaminophen, which will be useful in the event of any discomfort or slight fever, especially when you start vaccinations.
- Certain carryalls and portable cribs are very useful when going out, as well as a diaper bag that can also accommodate baby bottles and everything else you need when you're not at home. This is optional and you don't need to purchase it right away.

THE BABY CARRIAGE

Some suggestions:

- Above all, the baby carriage must be safe and strong. Other details to consider are price, ease of assembly, storage and handling, and appearance.
- The average price of a carriage is around $95, although there are some for as little as $20 and, at the other extreme, as high as $400. If you do not intend to have more children, consider buying a used carriage that is in good condition. (Better yet, borrow one!)
- The base of the carriage you choose should be wide, to avoid tipping in the event the baby leans out.
- Make sure it remains stable when you open it up, that it doesn't fold up unexpectedly, and that the brakes are easy to use and work well.
- It should have an awning or protective cover.
- Never leave your baby alone in its carriage, not even for a few seconds, even if he or she is sleeping comfortably.
- Remember that, if you hang heavy shopping bags from the carriage, it could tip over.

CHRISTIAN BACH
Actress (*Encandenados, Bajo un mismo rostro, Agua y aceite*) and soap opera producer (*Canaveral de passiones*)

My two pregnancies have been very good ones and for both I gained weight, but not more than sixteen pounds. I think the secret is not to think that, because we are pregnant, we need to gain huge amounts of weight, which gives us the excuse to eat everything we can think of and get fat. We must eat healthily, but also continue with our activities, and not regard ourselves as being sick. It is wonderful to continue doing as much exercise as possible, without harming ourselves. Attitude is very important in pregnancies; it is not good to become inactive or to think of yourself as incapable of doing anything.

My opinion is—and this is something my mother also says—that the child will fatten up outside his mother and not in his mother's tummy. You must eat well, but not so much as to give birth to very developed children.

Eating vegetables, protein, and a good diet helped me recover my figure quickly after giving birth. Breast-feeding babies also helps you get your figure back; I breast-fed both my sons for a month and a half. I not only think it's important for the child to receive this healthy nutrition from his mother, but it is also a way of bonding intimately and emotionally with them.

I became pregnant with my first son, Sebastián, fifteen days after I married Humberto, and I worked nonstop until the fifth month, on tour across the country with a theater production and shooting television programs.* After that, we went on our honeymoon (belated!) all across the Orient, and I returned to Mexico when I was already seven months pregnant. I think if the expectant mother has good experiences—like the ones I had on that trip, discovering other cultures in Thailand, China, and other countries—the baby also received them, because pregnancy is a very important sensorial moment, as much for the mother as for her baby.

*The Mexican actor and producer Humberto Zurita is Christian Bach's husband.

I did not feel ill on the trip, or after it, and continued with all kinds of activities after I returned. I think the only one who felt nauseated on the trip was Humberto! In addition, when I was nine months pregnant, I shot a commercial for dairy products, although they didn't show my whole body because I looked a little chubby.

With Sebastián, delivery was natural and quick. However, with the younger one, Emiliano—who is now three years old—a complication arose with the fact that, although the baby's head was already engaged, I still had no contractions; a week went by and still nothing. . . . The doctor induced my contractions, and still the baby would not be born. So, in order to avoid more serious problems (it seemed the heartbeats were weakening), I underwent a cesarean section. My surgery went extremely well, and I felt so good that I even wanted to attend a Michael Jackson concert for which I already had the tickets!

Chapter 7

THE ROLE OF THE FATHER AND SEXUAL RELATIONS

A SHARED PREGNANCY

THE FATHER'S CONCERNS

It would be unfair to say that the worries and discomforts, like the joys of pregnancy, belong exclusively to the mother. The majority of fathers feel that the problems of the pregnancy are theirs, too, even though they often don't know how to react to them.

Fortunately, the era when men felt they had done their duty as a father if their firstborn was a boy is long gone. It's not unusual to find men who prefer their first child to be a girl, recognizing that frequently girls are much more affectionate and closer to their fathers than to their mothers.

In other cases, the father decides that he will choose the child's name if it is a boy, while the mother is left to choose the girl's name. "My son will be a soccer player" or "I can't wait for the boy to be born, so I can take him fishing" are common expressions in fathers-to-be, which, although exaggerated, prove how excited they get at the prospect of having a child. This excitement can become the woman's best friend, by enabling her husband to be a real support to her during the difficult months that await them.

Did you know that there have been cases where future fathers have suffered morning sickness, difficulty sleeping, fatigue, cravings, and weight gain while their wives were pregnant? Surprisingly, as soon as the birth is over, these symptoms disappear.

Even though researchers have dedicated themselves to studying this phenomenon, they can't determine its cause. They think it must be due to an unconscious desire on the part of men to identify with their wives and to take part in the pregnancy process. It's not very common, but it's good for you to know about it, in case it happens to your partner.

The reality is that men's reactions to paternity, just like women's reactions regarding their pregnancies, manifest themselves in different ways in each individual. Many husbands feel an irresistible desire to protect their wives more during the months of pregnancy. If this is the case with your partner, don't reject it, even though you may be the most independent woman in the world and even if excessive protectiveness makes you uncomfortable. When the baby is born, those inclinations will leave him, and he will go back to treating you the way he did before.

Other husbands get jealous of the attention that their wife is getting from the rest of the family. They now feel that they've ceased to be the most important person in her life, since she has to divide her energy between her partner and the baby that is growing in her womb. "Before, you used to help choose the clothing *I* wore to work, but now you've only got time to get things ready for the *baby*," is a common complaint of jealous fathers-to-be. Be prepared to deal with your husband's jealousy, showing him proof of your love and attention. After all, up until this moment, he was the object of all your attention, and he needs time to get used to the fact that, in the future, he will have to share this attention with his child.

A typical concern of fathers during the months of pregnancy is whether they will be able to maintain the financial situation at home when the new member of the family arrives. And there are fathers who are horrified just to think that their children could be born with health problems, something that is also the main fear among many pregnant women.

In reality, your partner is concerned about the same things you are. The difference is that you dare to discuss your worries and anxieties while he keeps them inside because he's afraid of looking weak. Machismo comes into play even here!

Expecting only support and understanding from your husband would be a mistake for you. You should also be prepared to listen to him and pay attention to him when he decides to tell you what's on his mind or what's bothering him. Consider that, during the pregnancy, he is at a disadvantage with respect to you. You know that you're going through a natural process for a woman, and you are prepared to work with your doctor during the birth so that your baby is born without problems. You're the only one who can do that.

The delivery is a situation that is out of your husband's control. He has to be content with the role of spectator and can't even help you with so much as a push. Does that seem like a little thing? Up until now, he has been the indisputable hero of the household, the one who resolved all the difficult situations. Now, for the first time, a situation arises in which he can't take action and in which the solution doesn't lie in his hands.

MYTHS DURING PREGNANCY

- If the woman's womb is pointed, it's a boy; if it's round, it's a girl.
- If the baby moves a lot, it's a boy; if it's calmer, it's a girl.
- You have to eat for two.
- Firstborns always arrive late.
- A scare can induce birth immediately.
- If the mother has a scare, the baby will be born with a birthmark.
- If you dance during pregnancy, you will give birth ahead of schedule.
- More births take place during the full moon.
- If your mother had an easy birth, you will too.
- If you experience a lot of stomach acidity during pregnancy, the baby will be born with a lot of hair.
- It's bad luck to buy things for the baby before it's born.
- If you rub oil on your belly twice a day, you won't get stretch marks (lines due to stretching of the skin).
- Sexual relations during pregnancy will harm the baby.

This is why many men take refuge in their work when their wife's pregnancy reaches its final stage. Even though they appear to be indifferent, they are actually trying to avoid a problem that's out of their hands. By placing all their attention on their work, or a hobby, they avoid worrying about any complications during the delivery.

Knowing that these reactions are typical and very common in fathers-to-be will help you accept your husband the way he is, without demanding that he act differently or, even worse, labeling him a bad father. Remember that, in your case, it's what's in his heart that counts. It's important for the father-to-be not to feel like a mere spectator, but like an integral part of the pregnancy. An excellent idea is to ask him to go with you to a prenatal exercise program. He can learn the exercise routine and help you do it at home, and later, he can help you at the moment of the delivery, indicating the type of breathing you should do and how to relax between the contractions.

HOW TO COPE WITH A PREGNANT WOMAN

You never imagined that your wife would change so much during pregnancy. Before, she was always willing to make love with you whenever you wanted; she was always in a good mood; your sex life was excellent. Since she is a healthy woman, you don't recall having seen her sick, except for an insignificant cold.

Now everything has changed. You can't have coffee in bed in the morning because the smell of it makes her nauseated. She often seems tired and she rejects foods she used to love. Nevertheless, she wakes you up at one A.M. and asks you to order her a pizza with chili peppers, even though she used to hate the taste of chili. If you react in a negative way she bursts into tears, as though you had just insulted her mother. And if you start to caress her in bed the way you used to, from one moment to the next, she rolls over and starts snoring.

Ever since you got married, both of you planned to have several children. But now, given the way things are, you've reached the conclusion that this will be the first and last one.

Come on now, it's not that bad! After all, you're not the only man in the world who has gone through this, and the population on this planet keeps growing.

The first thing you have to do is arm yourself with a great deal of patience, because the pregnancy is just beginning. But, to reassure you, let me tell you that the nausea and vomiting stop around the fourth month. That's the good news. What about the bad news? Later other discomforts will appear. Don't worry about them. By then, you will have learned to cope with a pregnant woman.

Here are some suggestions that will help you.

- Show your wife how much you love her all the time, but don't hover over her as if she were sick. Although her condition is very special, pregnancy is not an illness.
- Make her understand that you still like her and that you still find her beautiful and attractive, even though her waistline is disappearing every day. Some women suffer the loss of their figure in silence, because they are afraid of not being attractive to their husbands anymore.
- Your wife is probably following the diet recommended by her doctor. Don't torture her by eating sweets and goodies in her presence when you know she can't join you.
- If she isn't willing to carry on the same sex life you had before, because she feels tired and lacks desire, don't force her. Substitute full sexual relations with other caresses, until after the first few weeks of the pregnancy. Generally speaking, she will then start to feel the same desire as before once this initial period is over.
- You might be like the majority of husbands who hate going shopping. But you should make an effort to go with her every so often to buy things for the baby. Your involvement will show her that you are interested in everything that concerns your future child.
- Don't smoke around your wife because your baby will also be exposed to the tobacco smoke by-products just as if your wife smoked. If you can't quit smoking, do it when your wife's not around.
- If you have to do home repairs in order to prepare the baby's room, try to have everything ready by the seventh month of pregnancy. Premature births are more common than you might imagine.
- Go with her to her prenatal exercise class, or ask her to teach you the routine so that you can assist her when she does it at home.
- Read books on prenatal child development. Being informed allows you to enjoy your baby's growth more and more each week, and to share it with your wife.
- Find out from the hospital whether you can be in the room during delivery. This will be a great source of moral support for her, and it will be a unique experience for you. Many fathers videotape the delivery of their child so they can preserve that very special moment.

MYTH: IF YOU DANCE DURING PREGNANCY, YOU WILL DELIVER AHEAD OF SCHEDULE

Unless you have had complications that require you to limit your physical activity significantly, if you like dancing, enjoy it! I'd like to point out the fact that this sentence does not specify what kind of dancing. Dancing salsa, cumbia, disco, rock, or slow dances is not the same. Pregnant women should avoid getting overtired. Avoid dancing for long periods without resting (this will also depend on your physical condition and your level of activity prior to pregnancy). You should avoid increasing your pulse rate over 140 beats per minute. Drink enough liquid to prevent dehydration and to keep your body temperature from rising above normal levels.

It's possible that you may have to rest more between dances as your pregnancy progresses, or that you dance more slow dances and fewer of the really fast ones.

SHARING THE BIRTH

No one will know better than your wife when it's time to go to the hospital. So, if you know that her water has broken and she's still taking her time having a shower, gathering her things, and then getting going, don't despair. Normally there are still several hours to go before your baby decides to be born.

Some hospitals allow the husband to accompany the pregnant woman during labor. If that is your wish, you will probably have to make the appropriate arrangements with the hospital. If this is not the case, you should wait in a waiting room until the baby is born.

Should you decide to stay with her until your baby is born, follow this advice:

- Keep her entertained so that she doesn't think about the contractions.
- Stay quiet and lower the lights so that she can rest, if that's what she chooses to do.
- Take a walk with her around the room, if she prefers to walk around.
- Make sure she is drinking liquids to prevent dehydration.

- When the contractions start to increase, help her to measure the time between them and assist her in doing the correct type of breathing.
- Remind her to rest between contractions.
- Offer her your hand or your arm to hold on to.
- Follow the instructions of the medical personnel.
- When the delivery is in process, encourage your wife to push when she needs to and to breathe in the way she was taught.
- Once the baby is born, hold him or her and share the joy of the moment with your wife.

Seventy-nine percent of fathers are present in the delivery room when their babies are born.

SOMEONE NEW AT HOME

Before the baby arrived, you and your wife were the ones who set the schedule. Now you'll have to adapt to the baby's schedule.

During the first few weeks of life, the baby will wake up several times during the night to be fed. This is your chance to play an important role in the caring of your child, something that was more difficult when the baby was in its mother's womb.

Raising a child should be both parents' job, not just the mother's. Learn to change diapers and to keep the baby clean and dry. This will be a good way to help your wife to rest and recover her energy if she is breast-feeding. If the baby is on formula, you might also learn to give him the bottle, taking turns so as to not leave the entire task to her. Besides, frequent contact with your son or daughter will help you get to know each other faster and help you distinguish the different types of cries: the ones due to hunger, the ones signaling a diaper change, and the ones when the baby wants to be picked up and comforted.

Once you are familiar with how to care for your baby, you will understand why your wife can't devote the same time to you as she did before. Nevertheless, this doesn't mean that you can't find a way to maintain your sense of intimacy. It requires planning and the taking advantage of those moments when the baby is asleep, which will be quite frequent during the first few months. In this way, you and your wife can renew your relationship with each other.

And, if you have a family member who is willing to stay with the baby now and then, take advantage of that in order to go out for a walk together or to go to a place you used to visit before. The baby's arrival doesn't have to create an emotional divide between the two of you. On the contrary, it should serve to further strengthen those ties between you.

> Some medical studies report that there is a slight increase in infertility in men who wear briefs or tight underwear.

> ## MYTH: SEXUAL RELATIONS DURING PREGNANCY HURT THE BABY
>
> When there is no problem or complication during pregnancy, sexual relations don't have to be avoided. Abstinence is recommended during certain periods of the pregnancy when there is a risk of abortion or a premature delivery. The baby is protected by the amniotic fluid in which it is floating. In some cases, in the ninth month, as the delivery date approaches, your doctor may recommend the use of a condom to decrease the risk of infection should the water break.
>
> My advice to you is: Listen to all these suggestions, find out which ones are true, laugh at the ones that are ridiculous, and forget about the rest.

SEX AND THE PREGNANT WOMAN

Don't believe anyone who tells you that sexual relations during pregnancy are harmful. Except in certain special cases where there is some problem with the pregnancy, abstinence is unnecessary. Moreover, we know that the contractions experienced by the pelvic muscles during the sexual act are exercises that strengthen them. What you can change are some of the positions you use, since certain positions that are uncomfortable for the pregnant woman, or that put pressure on her womb, are to be avoided.

Naturally, the situation is different with women who experience complications during pregnancy, including vaginal pain, or who run a risk of miscarriage, or who have had a series of previous miscarriages. In these cases, the doctor might recommend a period of abstinence from sexual relations during the delicate period of the first trimester.

There are cases, however, in which abstinence occurs for other reasons. There are men who, for fear of hurting their partner (even though this fear is unfounded), prefer to limit themselves to caresses and erotic games without penetration during this stage. There are also some women who are so concentrated on being mothers (or who feel so much physical discomfort) that they decide to give up sex altogether during those months. In this case, that decision should be respected, no matter whose it is.

> Forty-one percent of condoms in the United States are used by men and women between the ages of thirty-five and forty.

SEXUALITY DURING PREGNANCY

Your sexual behavior during pregnancy might really be disconcerting to your husband. That is why it is useful for both of you to know why you are reacting differently, if, up until that time, you have had a completely satisfactory sex life. It's possible that you may react differently to sexual stimuli during each stage of the pregnancy.

In general, during the first trimester pregnant women refuse sexual contact because they feel uncomfortable with their condition. It's impossible for you to feel like making love if you are nauseated all the time. You won't even let your husband caress your breasts if they are very tender. However, this attitude will change as those initial discomforts pass. You will discover how pleasurable it is to enjoy sex for its own sake and not as a reproductive function—you won't have to worry about using contraceptives.

Forget about the fear that penetration might harm the baby. He or she is having the time of his or her life, protected inside the amniotic sac. The baby won't notice anything except the mild pelvic contractions of orgasm. These will serve as precursors to the uterine contractions of birth; you will notice that, when these contractions stop, the baby will move around repeatedly, as if they had stimulated him or her as well. But don't worry, an orgasm will not rush delivery if your pregnancy is not at term yet.

Sometimes, especially during the third trimester, you might feel some cramps and back pain after having sexual intercourse. There is nothing to fear, because this is normal and is due to the congestion of the veins in the pelvic area during this stage of your pregnancy. You will also be surprised at how easy it is to enjoy multiple orgasms, something that might not have happened before. This takes place because the hormonal changes your body has undergone cause increased sensitivity in the vulvar region and increase the blood flow to the pelvis.

It's very important to communicate with your partner if you feel uncomfortable during sex. After all, this will last only a few months, and during this time, you can substitute other ways of showing love and affection.

YOUR PARTNER'S ATTITUDE

It's highly probable that, once your figure begins to show signs of the pregnancy, your husband will not express himself in intimate situations with the same impetuous passion you're used to. But before you blow this out of proportion, consider that he might be acting this way out of fear of hurting the baby. Actually, many men think they might hurt the baby during penetration, something that is absolutely false unless the pregnant woman has a natural predisposition toward miscarriages.

But if you help him understand, and work with him by trying to modify the positions in which you were previously used to making love, he will feel more confident. Each couple will find the position that is most comfortable for them and will modify it at different stages during the pregnancy. The most common positions are with both people lying on their side with vaginal entry from the side or rear in the spoon position; with the man on top of the woman, supporting himself with his hands so as to not rest his weight on her womb; and with the woman on top, but avoiding deep or violent penetration, which could be painful for her.

When you are in the final stages of pregnancy, your breasts may start to secrete colostrum each time that your husband stimulates them manually. If this bothers him, the answer would be not to touch them until they return to normal. But for the majority of men this is not a problem.

Don't be embarrassed to be naked with your husband. It may be that, when you see yourself in the mirror, you think you look horrible, with that enormous stomach and your belly button sticking out. However, men generally like it, and it excites them to see the new shape of their wife's body during the pregnancy. If a pregnant woman's body weren't beautiful, do you think so many Hollywood stars would have allowed their photographs to be taken (and published!) while they were pregnant?

WHAT YOU SHOULD AND SHOULDN'T DO

- Oral sex is allowed during pregnancy. However, during this time, you will experience an increase in vaginal secretions—which might bother your partner.

- If the doctor does not advise you to the contrary, the pelvic spasms brought on by orgasm will not cause any harm. If you don't feel like having sexual contact with penetration, you can achieve sexual satisfaction and intimacy through mutual manual stimulation.

- If you suspect that your partner might give you a sexually transmitted disease, ask him to use a condom each time you have intimate contact. This is the only way (although not 100 percent guaranteed) in which you can protect yourself and your baby.

- Although during the second and third trimesters of the pregnancy breast pain gradually disappears, your breasts are still highly sensitized, something that you have every right to enjoy when your partner caresses you and which you may find quite pleasurable.

- You should avoid vaginal penetration after engaging in anal penetration. This could cause a serious infection.

- Follow your instincts and common sense in choosing positions in which to have sex. Above all, protect your abdominal area.

VICTORIA RUFFO

Actress (*La fiera, Simplemente María,*
Pobre niña rica, Abrázame muy fuerte, La madrastra)

During the first month of my pregnancy with my first son, Jose Eduardo, I felt a lot of nausea, dizziness, and irritability. On more than one occasion I felt I would die, but I never felt that I didn't want to be pregnant! On the contrary, the thought that I would soon have that little piece of flesh in my arms that I could care for and protect made me happier and more expectant than ever. Also, I felt very sleepy. Aside from the normal eight hours, I would find ways to take naps all day long, half hour or even an hour.

Normally, my blood pressure is low, but due to the pregnancy, it would drop something crazy. And, of course, this frightened me a lot. My only craving was for avocados. I gained ten kilos, which is not too much, and because I'm so skinny, they looked great on me. Mentally is where I really felt the discomforts of pregnancy the most. I would become very anxious, thinking about how I would face my responsibility of educating, bathing, feeding my child. "What if I can't get any more work . . . what will we eat? Where will we live?" I'd ask myself.

I took my preparatory course, but at the time, I was so scared that it didn't help very much, because theory has a lot to do with practice. The situation and discomfort didn't improve very much during my second pregnancy.

But the worst thing was that I had to undergo a cesarean. Since I'd never had surgery, I was not only scared but truly terrified to think that I was so narrow that the only way I could give birth was by means of a cesarean section.

After all of these things, I think I am the least likely to give a first-timer any advice. But I can tell her to face her pregnancy as the greatest and most beautifully satisfying event a woman can have.

Chapter 8

THE FIRST TRIMESTER

The signs and symptoms we have mentioned vary with each woman. In fact, the same woman may feel differently at different times.

THE FIRST MONTH: CHANGES IN THE MOTHER

PHYSICAL

In the initial phase, during the first few days following conception, the pregnant woman rarely, if ever, realizes she is pregnant. The first month almost always passes unnoticed; however, this is the stage in which gestation begins. At this point, the being that is forming is known as an embryo. It isn't until the third month that it is called a fetus. The following changes may take place in the first month:

- Possible appearance of dark patches on the skin
- Increase in breast tenderness
- Changes in the color of the gums (which turn red)

So, starting with the first month, once she knows she is pregnant, the future mother must start to take certain precautions, such as ceasing to drink alcoholic beverages, quitting smoking, and not taking any medicine (even if it is sold without a prescription) without consulting her doctor.

PHYSIOLOGICAL

- Dizziness, fatigue
- Light vaginal bleeding
- Possible nausea or vomiting in the morning due to disturbances of the digestive system
- Heartburn or a burning sensation in the stomach area
- Aversion to certain foods
- Loss of appetite
- Possible increase in the amount of saliva
- Cramps

PSYCHOLOGICAL

- Tension due to worries related to the pregnancy
- Sudden changes in mood, irritability
- Lack of willpower, physical lethargy
- Doubts, uncertainty
- A tendency to become isolated
- Difficulty concentrating and remaining concentrated, self-absorption
- Anxiety
- Depression for no apparent reason
- Ambivalent feelings, confusion between joy and doubt
- Worry about one's financial future following the birth
- Feelings of loneliness
- Joy and enthusiasm at the news of the pregnancy

MYTHS BASED ON MAGIC AND FOLKLORE

- If a pregnant woman sleeps during the day, her child will be born with protruding eyelids.
- If a pregnant woman chews gum, the baby's palate will harden and his gums will become thick. This will not allow the baby to breast-feed and he will die of starvation.
- If a pregnant woman eats tamales that have stuck to the pan, the child will stick to her womb and not be able to come out at the time of delivery.
- If a pregnant woman sees people being hanged, the child will become entangled in its umbilical cord.
- Sexual intercourse is advised after the first trimester, so that the child will grow properly; if he is lacking that source of energy, he will be weak and sickly. But when the womb is already rounded, sexual intercourse is forbidden because the child will emerge soiled upon delivery, as though he had been bathed in cornstarch, or he will become stuck to the womb and the birth will be long and painful.

THE SECOND MONTH: CHANGES IN THE MOTHER

PHYSICAL

During the second month of gestation, generally speaking, you visit the doctor to verify your suspicions (following the absence of menstruation and certain mild discomforts) that you're pregnant. The following changes are typical:

- Mild swelling of the hands, feet, and/or face
- Hardening and increase in the size of the breasts and nipples
- Slight increase in weight. In many cases this is due to anxiety. Women who are overweight before the pregnancy are advised to be careful not to gain too much more; those who are below their normal weight are advised to try to gain weight

at the beginning of the pregnancy, especially if they suffer from vomiting and nausea. The weight lost due to those factors is quickly regained.

- Broadening of the hips due to pelvic expansion
- Change in color of the nipple and the areola. These areas may turn darker, and the areola glands may appear more prominent.
- Light irritation of the gums, accompanied by inflammation
- Softer and more brittle fingernails
- Darkening of skin color on some areas of the body, perhaps in the form of a line between the belly button and the pubic area, or on the face

PHYSIOLOGICAL

- Difficulty sleeping, insomnia. During the first months of pregnancy you feel an irresistible urge to sleep, although soon, during the final stages, difficulty sleeping will be a very common problem. The movements of the fetus in the womb may cause insomnia; when this occurs, a change in position may help.
- Compression of the bladder due to the increase in size of the uterus and the weight of the fetus. This creates pressure that increases the desire to urinate frequently.
- Swelling of the feet. Veins may look more prominent.
- Irritation of the skin and an itchy sensation throughout the body
- Mineral deficiency. This could contribute to the lack of calcium in the bones, to anemia, and to skin discoloration. Your doctor will evaluate your diet and advise you on which vitamins and minerals to take.
- Acidity, especially in the morning
- Constipation
- Gas, indigestion
- Muscle and joint pains
- Headaches, migraines
- Pain in the back and waist. As the pregnancy progresses, your body's posture will change to compensate for the weight and volume of the uterus.
- Cravings. These might appear during the first trimester and may last throughout the pregnancy.
- You may notice an excess in the production of saliva. Generally this symptom disappears in the second trimester, but it could last throughout the pregnancy.

- Nausea and vomiting in the morning. Nausea generally appears at the third week and disappears around the fourth month. It occurs more frequently in the morning or during periods of fasting, and disappears after breakfast. If it persists, you should consult your doctor so that he or she can determine if there is another cause.

PREVENTING NAUSEA*

In the morning
- If nausea occurs in the morning, have breakfast in bed before getting up and remain lying down.
- Eat toast or soda crackers.
- Drink hot tea, such as chamomile or licorice.

During the day
- Divide your typical three meals into smaller amounts and eat several small meals throughout the day.
- Avoid greasy foods or foods that are difficult to digest.
- If solid food causes more problems than liquid, drink lots of fluids when you experience nausea and eat solid food when you don't feel nauseated.
- Consume only liquids at one meal and then only solid food at another.
- Drink sips of carbonated soda. Choose one that doesn't contain caffeine.
- Grate ginger, a natural remedy for nausea, over vegetables or other foods.
- Suck on a freshly cut lemon. This might cause heartburn.
- Avoid things that induce nausea, such as certain odors, movements, or sounds.
- Avoid getting overheated and sweating profusely, which could contribute to nausea.

*Don't take any medicine for nausea that has not been prescribed by your doctor.

(continued on next page)

PREVENTING NAUSEA *(continued)*

At night

■ Make dinner simple and light. Avoid eating large amounts or foods that are difficult to digest (greasy, seasoned food).

■ Take your vitamins with food at night if this is the time when you feel least nauseated. Some doctors recommend taking more vitamin B_6 (around 50 micrograms extra) in order to lessen nausea.

PSYCHOLOGICAL

- Anxiety about the loss of your figure. It is inevitable that pregnancy will radically alter your physical shape; however, you should remember that these physical and psychological changes are perfectly normal and temporary and that, for the time being, you don't have to turn this into a tragedy. Try to accept, enjoy, and adapt to your new condition. Remaining calm will help not only your physical and mental health, but also the health of your baby.
- Irritability
- Uncontrollable, unprovoked crying followed by laughter and joy
- Concern over the different physical and psychological changes that are occurring
- Nightmares (almost always associated with the baby and the delivery)
- The need for attention during this period. Without realizing it, you have become very vulnerable and are demanding to be spoiled and taken care of all the time.
- Fears, expectations, possible absentmindedness
- Difficulty in focusing your attention and your concentration on daily chores
- Creating fantasies with the image of the child you are expecting; silent conversations with your future child

THE THIRD MONTH: CHANGES IN THE MOTHER

PHYSICAL

- Weight gain
- Increase in the size of the uterine cavity upon stretching of uterine ligaments
- Broadening of the cheekbones, nose, and mouth
- Continuing increase in the size of the breasts
- Swelling of the hands and feet
- Increase in the size of the abdomen
- Appearance of stretch marks on the skin

PHYSIOLOGICAL

- Headaches. Sometimes these are due to changes in arterial pressure.
- Possible urinary infections
- Possible loss of sex drive. With some exceptions, a couple may have sexual intercourse during pregnancy. However, there are a host of psychological barriers that could be inhibiting. One of them is believing that the uterine contractions produced during orgasm can cause a miscarriage or a premature birth. Unless your doctor has asked you to refrain from sexual intercourse because of a particular problem in your case, there is no need to do so. Obviously you don't have to have sex if you don't feel like it.
- Change in sleep patterns

PSYCHOLOGICAL

- Emotional states, including hopes, fears, and concern for the physical well-being of the baby
- Interest in learning about giving birth and making postpartum plans
- Joyful feelings when in the presence of small children
- A desire to communicate in a more direct way with your baby—caressing your belly, talking lovingly to him or her

MYTH: BIRTHS INCREASE DURING THE FULL MOON

It is also said that lunatics emerge during the full moon. Scientific studies do not support either theory 100 percent. Some people say that when the barometric pressure is lowered such as during the full moon, a snowstorm, or a hurricane, the force of gravity causes one's water to break, which is why there are more births on those days.

Perhaps conception increases on those days as well. Yet this would have nothing to do with the force of gravity. . . . The full moon also has been associated with romance. . . . I'll let you draw your own conclusions.

THE BABY'S DEVELOPMENT

Around twenty-one days after the last menstruation, the fertilized egg adheres to the wall of the uterus. For the first eight weeks it is known as an embryo; then it is called a fetus. In the first month, it measures about one-quarter to one-half inch and has a cleft, or canal, that will subsequently become the nervous system. It has protrusions that will later develop into vertebrae, ribs, and muscles in the torso. The baby's digestive system is beginning to form.

In the beginning of the first trimester, the internal organs start to develop, among them the heart and the cardiovascular system (which makes this a delicate stage for cardiac malformations). At one end, a knob that will become the head (now containing a rudimentary brain) appears. Beginning with small stumps, the arms and legs slowly start to develop and stretch out, and the transparent skull allows us to see the baby's brain.

Around the sixth week, twenty-five little cubes appear in a line down the middle of the spine. These are the future vertebrae (increasing quickly in number until they reach forty-one). On its head, which now begins to separate a little from the neck, you can see the curves of the ears, chin, and neck. At the end of the first trimester, the lips take shape, and tooth sockets and buds are forming in the jawbones. By this time, the nostrils have completely formed.

By the eighth week, the embryo measures one and one-eighth inches. The head and torso have straightened out, the fingers on the hands appear with interdigital membranes, and the toes also begin to elongate. It is *important* to remember that during this entire time (especially until the eighth week, more or less)—while the embryo is developing—any accident, trauma, or infection that you suffer could cause permanent damage to your baby's central nervous system, as well as any of its future organs.

Starting with the ninth week, the development of the fetus is focused on the growth and maturity of the tissues and organs that started to form during the embryonic stage. Now the fetus measures one and one-quarter inches in length and weighs around one-half ounce. The first signs of sexual differentiation appear—that is, the factors determining whether it will be a boy or a girl—and the digestive system is now capable of producing movement and contractions.

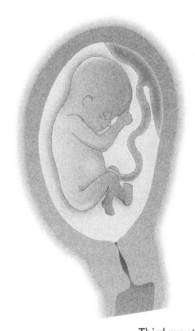

Third month

Around the end of the first trimester, the baby's head occupies a third of the total body, and the bones begin to harden, as do fingernails and skull. Although you don't feel it yet, by this stage the fetus is already moving.

The embryo, and subsequently the fetus, is protected throughout the pregnancy by the amniotic sac, a membrane filled with amniotic fluid that the baby floats in. The umbilical cord connects the baby to the placenta, the organ that is attached to the uterus and that allows an exchange between the mother's bloodstream and the baby's. It is the fetus's life-support system. The placenta nourishes the fetus, giving it food, antibodies against disease, and oxygen; taking away its waste products; and producing certain hormones that allow the pregnancy to continue. By the ninth month, the placenta will weigh about one and a half pounds.

ANGÉLICA RIVERA
Actress (*La dueña, Angela, Huracán,
Sin pecado concebido, Mariana de la noche*)

My first daughter, Angélica Sofía, weighed 3 kilos 300 grams and measured 51 centimeters at birth. While pregnant, I had cravings for pastries and desserts, but avoided eating them, not so that I would not lose my figure, but because I thought they would not be good for the baby. If I was not concerned about interrupting my career (which was, at the time, at a peak) in order to fulfill my womanhood and bring a child into the world, much less did I care about losing my figure! The first few months I felt very sleepy and, in order to have a healthy baby, I quit smoking.

Many of my friends suggested I have an ultrasound to find out the baby's sex, but neither my husband nor I agreed to it. We always believed that the fact that the baby would be a surprise made the joy of the birth more complete. Even though the doctors did everything they could so that I would have a natural childbirth, it was not possible, and it was necessary to perform a cesarean section. When I held my little girl in my arms, I was overcome with emotion. I had no problem breast-feeding her myself, and that makes me confident that she will grow up healthy and strong. I only gained nine kilos, which I lost almost completely within the first month after giving birth.

Chapter 9

THE SECOND TRIMESTER

Please remember that not all the signs or symptoms that I mention appear in all women. Some appear at different times even in the same woman.

THE FOURTH MONTH: CHANGES IN THE MOTHER

PHYSICAL

- The abdomen keeps on growing, as do the breasts.
- The legs swell and the veins of the abdomen and legs (or the varicose veins, if you have them, in the legs) become more noticeable as your weight increases.
- Facial features change slightly.
- The weight of the abdomen tilts the spine forward, arching it.
- Texture of the hair changes, becoming a lot drier.

PHYSIOLOGICAL

- The amount of blood and fluids in the body increases.
- The volume of amniotic fluid increases.

- You may develop an iron, calcium, magnesium, or zinc deficiency (which your doctor will help to prevent by counseling you on your diet and by prescribing prenatal vitamins and minerals in pill form).
- You may notice a slight shortness of breath.
- You may notice swelling as a result of fluid retention.
- Some women develop allergies to certain things in the environment, to certain plants, to certain animals and/or dust, etc.
- You could notice a thick, white, milky secretion from your breasts.
- Irritation may develop on the skin of the face, arms, and legs.
- Nausea and vomiting usually disappear or decrease.
- You may feel increasingly sleepy or drowsy during the day.
- There is an increased risk of sugar levels rising in the blood, which could cause diabetes.
- You may experience cystitis, a burning sensation when urinating. (This usually suggests a bladder infection.)
- You may have frequent nasal or ear congestion, and possible nosebleeds.
- You could notice light bleeding from your gums when you brush your teeth.
- You may develop hemorrhoids, in some cases with bleeding after a bowel movement.
- You could experience constipation and abdominal distension caused by gas.

PSYCHOLOGICAL

- You may feel unconscious hostility toward those close to you who don't respond to your constant need for attention. (You may feel irritable and display this symptom within the first three months.)
- Some women feel frustrated that they cannot wear maternity clothes because they still haven't gained enough weight, while their regular clothes don't fit anymore—they are too tight.
- You become extroverted, gregarious. You seek contact with nature (the beach, parks, lakes, etc.) and the company of other pregnant women and mothers.

MYTH: IF YOUR MOTHER EXPERIENCED AN EASY DELIVERY, YOURS WILL ALSO BE EASY

It's true that inheritance plays an important role in the size of the pelvis and certain other physical and mental characteristics that may contribute to the degree of difficulty of the delivery. However, there are many other factors that determine how easy or difficult it will be: the baby's position and size, the mother's nutrition, certain habits the mother may have such as smoking, exercising, etc.

THE FIFTH MONTH: CHANGES IN THE MOTHER

PHYSICAL

- Stretch marks on the skin of the abdomen and arms
- Rapid increase in weight
- Noticeable tilting of spine and shoulders
- Continued swelling of limbs, especially feet and hands
- Aching of the back and the spine
- Swollen varicose veins
- Body aches due to bad posture while sleeping
- Detection of fetal movements

PHYSIOLOGICAL

- Increase in vaginal discharge, which is thick and white
- Sweating
- Numbness in the arms and legs
- Sudden changes in body temperature
- Aching of the head and pelvis
- Increased pulse rate, sometimes accompanied by palpitations

PSYCHOLOGICAL

- Impatience and irritability, but mood swings are less intense
- Anxiety
- Concern over the baby's normal development and the pregnancy
- Adaptation to the physiological changes happening in your body
- Excitement and motivation about the pregnancy and the baby
- Awareness of the need to exercise, walk, swim, squat, etc.

Fifty-two percent of the men who have been U.S. presidents were the firstborn sons in their family. Twenty-one of the first twenty-three U.S astronauts were the eldest son of the family.

THE SIXTH MONTH: CHANGES IN THE MOTHER

PHYSICAL

- Weight increase continues, as does the widening of the hips.
- Breasts are tender, resulting from an increase in size.
- Blotches and stretch marks on the skin continue.
- Gums bleed.
- Back and spine ache due to the weight of the abdomen and the tilting of the spine (sciatica).

PHYSIOLOGICAL

- Fluctuating blood pressure
- Itching all over the body
- Indigestion accompanied by distention due to gas
- Nasal and ear congestion
- Constant thirst, a need to consume large quantities of fluids
- Constipation
- Aching joints, hands, arms, and knees (however, it is not recommended that pregnant women take aspirin, especially during the last three months before the baby's arrival)
- Fatigue

PSYCHOLOGICAL

- Forgetfulness, difficulty concentrating, apathy
- Anxiety, which provokes the need to eat certain foods (cravings), which in turn may produce weight gain
- Frequent dreams about the coming baby, the delivery, the home. Occasionally, you may have nightmares related to the delivery and the fetus.

STATISTICS ON PREGNANCY

- The United States has twice as many teenage pregnancies as any other industrialized nation in the world. More than 80 percent of these pregnancies in minors are unplanned.
- Three of every five adult women, and four of every five teenagers, have no idea as to when they are most likely to get pregnant. The majority of these women do not know that the highest risk of getting pregnant is when sexual intercourse takes place fourteen days after the first day of menstruation (when the menstrual cycle is a regular twenty-eight-day cycle).
- Black women are 25 percent more prone to multiple births than white women.
- Every woman has a 2 percent chance of giving birth to twins . . . or more (multiple births).

THE BABY'S DEVELOPMENT

In the third and fourth months of pregnancy, the fetus grows from approximately four to seven inches and from one to eight ounces. The face is defined: Eyes, mouth, nose, and ears are almost completely formed. The eyelids are contracted, but still closed. The mouth opens and closes. The neck moves in all directions.

Arms and legs have lengthened and the gastrointestinal system is developed, allowing the fetus to swallow the amniotic fluid (which is the liquid that surrounds and protects

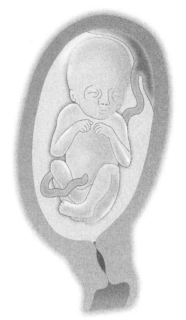

Fourth month

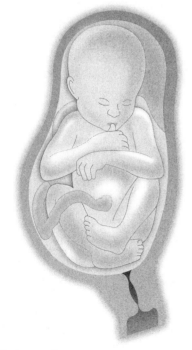

Sixth month

it). The liver, pancreas, and salivary glands are actively functioning, while the spinal cord is completely structured.

At the beginning of the fifth month, hair, eyebrows, and the nails of the toes begin to appear, and a very fine down covers the body. The future baby grimaces, frowns, and blinks. The mother begins to notice fetal movements within her abdomen; she feels the gentle tapping the fetus makes with its hands and feet. In this phase, the heart rate is at one hundred forty beats per minute. From now on, the infant alternates between sleep and waking periods.

Between the fifth and seventh months of pregnancy, the fetus grows in weight from one to three pounds, and in length from nine to seventeen inches. In its body, which is now more proportioned, the sebaceous glands begin to function, secreting an oily substance (vernix caseosa), which forms a protective layer that blankets the fetal skin until the moment of birth. This fine layer replaces the fine down that previously covered its body.

The knees remain stuck to the abdomen and the arms folded on the chest, although, generally, their movements are more vigorous. The nose and nasal orifices are well defined; the eyelids separate and the eyes open partially. The ears grow and the neck stretches; the fetus begins to suck a finger. This is the phase when the mother may experience her baby's hiccups, which feel somewhat like a heartbeat in her lower abdomen.

As a result of the development of the senses, the fetus is capable of hearing toward the end of this trimester. Not only does it constantly hear the sounds coming from its mother's heart and other organs, but also its own heartbeat and the noises and sounds of the outside world. Some outside sounds are pleasant and comforting, like its parents' voices. Others are startling, such as all loud, sharp, or boisterous noises. The fetus is also sensitive to light and reacts when its mother's abdomen is exposed to the sun.

Even though the fetus already has all of its organs in a fairly developed stage (between the fifth and sixth months), it would run the risk of dying within hours if it were born at this time, because its respiratory system is still immature.

NATALIA ESPERÓN

Actress (*Agujetas color de rosa, Por un beso, La esposa virgen*)

During my pregnancy, I got strong cravings to eat green tamales, *mole,* and everything that was typical Mexican food. I gained eighteen kilos, but after the postpartum quarantine, I made sure I lost all the weight with diets and exercise routines.

Although a lot of people told us that ultrasound was not a 100 percent sure way of knowing the baby's sex and we could be disappointed, we took a chance. And we won; it was a girl! Her name is Natalia, like mine, and she weighed 2 kilos 500 grams and was 50 centimeters long at birth. I feel that being a mother at such a young age (I'm twenty-one) is an advantage, because it will allow me to have a better relationship with my daughter.

The worst thing about my pregnancy was the cesarean section I had to undergo. I was very scared when I arrived, because there never fails to be somebody telling you it's a terrible moment and I felt I would die. However, the doctors were excellent, and I hardly felt anything. Moreover, when you see your little one all wide-eyed and moving its feet and hands, you forget everything. . . .

Among the most vivid memories this first pregnancy left me—since we have thought of having two or three babies more but will wait for three years—is seeing my husband chatting to calm me down and later to find out he was the one who cut the umbilical cord.

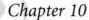

Chapter 10

THE THIRD TRIMESTER

THE SEVENTH MONTH: CHANGES IN THE MOTHER

PHYSICAL

- Weight gain due to the increased volume of fluids in the body
- Further imbalance in the posture. The shoulders and hips tilt toward the front or the sides.
- Discomfort in the lower abdomen and backache
- Continued dilation of varicose veins

PHYSIOLOGICAL

- Slight shortness of breath. Breathing becomes irregular and may produce a frequent feeling of suffocation.
- Increased fetal activity
- Increase in the amount of vaginal discharge
- Constipation, indigestion, and distention due to gas
- Hemorrhoids

- Accumulation of fluids in the limbs (during the daytime, in the legs and feet)
- Change in the color of the urine due to the presence of glucose (sugar) or of infections. This is not normal and requires treatment.

PSYCHOLOGICAL

- Psychological preparations for the delivery
- Mixed feelings of fear and joy
- "Prenatal fantasies," which last longer. You imagine your baby and the delivery while paying less attention to the social and family environment.
- Need for loving physical contact, hugs, caresses, etc.

THE EIGHTH MONTH: CHANGES IN THE MOTHER

PHYSICAL

- Continuation of some of the discomforts that appeared earlier, many of them due to your weight and to physical changes in your motor system, meaning your bones, muscles, and joints. The backache worsens.
- Feeling of tautness in the groin and pelvic area
- Heaviness in the pubic area. Some positions prove painful.
- Increase in the size of the uterus, which constricts the diaphragm (the muscle that separates the thorax from the abdomen), causing abdominal pain and possible protrusion of your navel
- Sensation of shortness of breath, even though your breathing rate does not vary

MYTH: IF YOU EXPERIENCE A LOT OF HEARTBURN DURING PREGNANCY, THE BABY WILL BE BORN WITH A LOT OF HAIR

Heartburn is caused by the reflux of stomach acid to the esophagus. The esophagus is the connecting tube between the mouth and the stomach. A tiny muscle between the esophagus and the stomach normally keeps the acid from flowing back into the esophagus. Hormones such as progesterone diminish the strength of this muscle during pregnancy, allowing the acid flow. In addition, the growing womb pushes other organs within the abdomen, including the stomach. This, too, may cause heartburn. This condition is more frequent in the second and third trimesters of pregnancy.

Now . . . the association between heartburn and hair on the baby has no scientific basis. I have had patients who have not suffered heartburn and have given birth to babies with a lot of hair, others who suffered from intense heartburn who gave birth to babies who were bald. Neither is the amount of hair associated with spicy food or chilis. Even though there are people who believe that putting chili on their scalp will grow more hair, in reality it is digested in the stomach. By the time chili eaten by a mother-to-be reaches the baby in the womb, it is unrecognizable as chili.

By the way, I am not suggesting or recommending that chili be used on the scalp.

PHYSIOLOGICAL

- Extreme sleepiness
- Possible dizziness, headaches, or feeling of faintness
- Continued and heavier vaginal discharge
- Continued indigestion, heartburn, and constipation
- Varied heart rate, possibly reaching as much as ten heartbeats per minute over your normal count (slight tachycardia)

- Increase in the blood flow to the uterus
- Increased fetal activity
- Increased retention of fluids, especially in the legs, particularly at the end of the day

PSYCHOLOGICAL

- Increased fear of a long labor with complications
- The increased wish to see the end of the pregnancy

THE NINTH MONTH: CHANGES IN THE MOTHER

PHYSICAL

- Continued and increased vaginal discharge, with mucus and, occasionally, blood spotting
- Soreness of the breasts, back, and pelvis, increasing in severity as the moment of labor and delivery approaches
- Dilated varicose veins in the legs

PHYSIOLOGICAL

- Pain and alarm at the possibility of "false labor" due to contractions becoming more intense and, sometimes, painful
- Quick, irregular contractions
- Diarrhea, in many cases uncontrollable
- Rupture of the membranes, your "water breaks." (This means labor is imminent.)
- Constipation
- Heartburn, acidity in the stomach, abdominal distention due to gas
- Hemorrhoids
- Dizziness, feeling faint, and/or headaches
- Nasal congestion with occasional nosebleed and ear congestion
- Redness of the gums, occasionally with bleeding
- Leg cramps
- Difficulty sleeping
- Increased frequency of urination

P S Y C H O L O G I C A L

- Enthusiasm and joy on the one hand, feelings of fear on the other
- Anxiety and distortions in the perception of time
- Relief to know the pregnancy is reaching term
- The joy of anticipation

HOW MANY BABIES ARE BORN IN EACH MONTH?

According to Tom Heymann's book *Unofficial Census in the United States*, more babies are born in the United States during some months than in others. The following is the ranking, from most to least:

1. September
2. March
3. May
4. January and August

5. February
6. July and December
7. June
8. April

9. November
10. October

THE BABY'S DEVELOPMENT

During the final three months, the fetus basically grows in size, since its body and the organs of its senses (hearing, sight, smell, taste, and touch) are fully developed and must simply mature.

Between the sixth and seventh months, it measures between eleven and seventeen inches and can weigh anywhere from one and one-half to three pounds. The eyes are completely open, but the pupils are still covered by a membrane. The nervous system has matured considerably.

The lungs function for breathing and the fetus can inhale and exhale, rhythmically controlling the breathing and temperature of its body. The bone marrow begins producing red blood cells, and the gastrointestinal system starts producing certain substances. Meconium appears, which is, essentially, the first feces produced by the fetus.

In this phase the fetus possesses almost all of its neurons. The neurons establish relationships between the nerve centers, which by this time are already complex. The infant's reflexes—moving of arms and legs and turning over—have matured, and muscle strength is greater. The seven-month-old fetus is ready for birth, but its condition is still fragile and it doesn't have sufficient weight or energy to face the outside world.

Between seven and eight months, its weight is about two and one-half to six pounds and it measures fourteen to eighteen inches. The stomach, intestines, and kidneys function as they will in the future, and all of the most important organs are ready.

Cerebral activity is apparent. At the end of the third trimester, the membrane that covered the pupils disappears, allowing the eyes to respond to intense light. In this phase, the fetus should adopt the cephalic (head down) position. This does not always occur; some adopt other positions such as breech, feet first, face forward, etc. The cephalic position is the most appropriate, making it easy for the fetus to enter the birth canal.

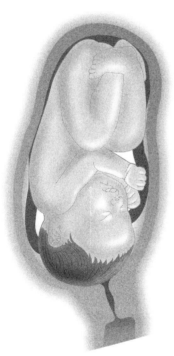

Eighth to ninth month

Between eight and nine months, the fetus now measures approximately sixteen to twenty-two inches and weighs four to ten pounds. The future child is completely formed; he or she makes fists, has a sense of taste, and shows a protruding thorax. In the case of boys, testicles have come down from the scrotum. As it has increased in size and weight, the baby moves less frequently but with more strength and, toward the end of the month, is ready to be born.

In the ninth month, the baby adopts the delivery position. The umbilical cord and the womb, along with the baby's body, form one compact mass. At this moment, the fetus occupies his mother's abdomen almost entirely. It is relaxed; breathing is gentler and slower. It continues to respond to vibrations, light, and sound, which is a positive sign.

Several tests will be done during this month, such as an ultrasound to measure the fetus's motor response, the amount of available amniotic fluid, and the frequency of the fetus's heartbeats.

ALEJANDRA ÁVALOS
Actress (*El padre Gallo, Morir dos veces,
Soñadoras, Apuesta por un amor*) and singer

Without knowing why, I became addicted to lemon during my pregnancy, which is something that I hadn't liked very much before that. You won't believe all the things that happened to me: I craved typical Mexican foods, especially the ones with very hot spices. I would become terribly thirsty, I needed to go to the bathroom all the time, I had headaches, insomnia, I would fall into depressions . . . I became unbearable!

My daughter, Valentina, was born by cesarean section. This decision was made because my pelvic cavity turned out to be very narrow and the baby presented itself face forward. I asked the doctors to give me a saddle block so I wouldn't feel any pain, because I wanted to concentrate on the music of Mozart, which I specifically chose for that day. In the morning, I thought that creating in my womb a being that had my blood and my flesh was the closest thing to a miracle. My daughter's first cry is something I will remember my whole life, and that my husband was brave enough to cut the umbilical cord filled me with emotions that are hard to explain. I gained thirteen kilos with this pregnancy, lost seven with the delivery, and so far, six months later, I have not been able to shed the rest.

The fact that my mother breast-fed me, or maybe because I was given the opportunity, I decided to breast-feed Valentina. She's a glutton and I have to feed her every two and a half hours. This is very exhausting, especially when it has to be done at night, or early morning. But my reward, aside from seeing her satisfied, is watching my husband burp her and change her diaper. For the time being we want to devote ourselves entirely to Valentina because, at this age, children are so defenseless that they require a lot of care. My advice to first timers, especially Latino mothers, is to get close to your mother during your pregnancy. She will always know what to do.

Chapter 11

THE BIG EVENT

GENERAL ADVICE FOR YOUR LAST WEEKS OF PREGNANCY

- Whenever you can, raise your feet. (This way you will avoid swelling in the ankles, and varicose veins.)
- Go to the doctor once a week.
- Try not to lie on your back, since this could cause you discomfort or shortness of breath.
- Buy brassieres that are designed for nursing, if you plan to nurse your baby. These will be the most comfortable.
- Buy everything you need for the baby's basic needs.
- Pack the suitcase you will be taking to the hospital when you deliver.

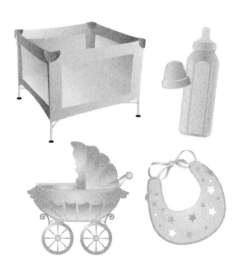

- Keep the pantry stocked with foods that are easy to prepare so that you won't have to worry about that when you come home from the hospital.
- Ask your doctor to arrange a visit to the birthing center or maternity ward of the hospital where you will deliver.
- Rest and relax as much as possible. It's common for you to have difficulty sleeping during this period and to feel especially tired.
- Try to avoid as much as possible doing things that make you impatient or upset. Stay calm and devote yourself to doing things related to the baby that please you (like knitting some clothes for him or her), reading light and pleasant material, or practicing your birthing exercises, etc.

THE DELIVERY

This is divided into three stages:

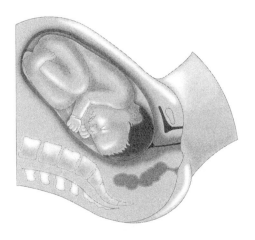

- First stage: The prebirth, or labor, which includes everything from the initial regular contractions that make the cervix begin to stretch and open up until the cervix is completely dilated, thus allowing space for the baby to exit through the vagina (the birth canal).

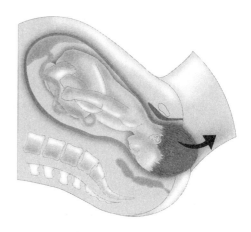

- Second stage: The birth itself, which culminates in the emergence of the baby and his or her birth.

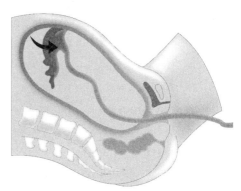

- Third stage: The emergence of the placenta after the baby is born.

WHAT ARE WE GOING TO NAME THE BABY?

These are some beautiful names for boys and girls that follow our Hispanic-American tradition and have been quite popular in recent years.

GIRLS		BOYS	
Alejandra	Marisa	Alejandro	Gabriel
Carolina	Patricia	Carlos	José
Fernanda	Sandra	Daniel	Luis Miguel
Isabella	Valeria	Diego	Paco
Mariana	Verónica	Eduardo	Rodrigo
		Emilio	Santiago

FIRST STAGE OF THE DELIVERY

PREBIRTH (EARLY PHASE)

The intermittent and painless contractions you have been feeling during the last months will gradually become more and more painful until the end of the ninth month (they will closely resemble typical menstrual cramps). But these are only false alarms, and you should learn to distinguish them from "real" contractions. These are the ones that signal the imminent birth and are the result of abrupt movements in the uterine muscles, which are contracting in order to open the cervix in preparation for the baby's exit through the birth canal. You should measure the interval between contractions so as to be able to tell when they are occurring with greater frequency. The main characteristics of real labor contractions include the following:

- They are painful and increase in intensity over time, but this pain disappears between each contraction.
- They come according to a fixed rhythm, that is, at first they occur about every half hour, and as the delivery draws nearer, they occur more frequently and at regular intervals.
- They are not interrupted (like the "false alarms") once they start.
- In the beginning each one lasts some fifteen seconds, but later they last longer, although no more than fifty to sixty seconds.

No one, not even the most experienced physician, can tell you the exact day that the baby is due. This means that you should be prepared several days ahead of the approximate date they have given you. And when we say "prepared," we mean ready to rush to the hospital at any time, without having to get things together or wait for anything.

You have probably heard, on radio or television, of extraordinary cases of women who deliver in a taxi or in the ambulance on the way to the hospital, but these cases are the exceptions. The first symptoms generally appear several hours ahead of the baby's arrival. However, there's always the possibility that you will deliver faster than you expected. If you are home alone, call someone you know immediately so he or she can take you to the hospital, or, if you prefer, call a taxi or an ambulance.

Even if there is a long time between contractions, leave your house in plenty of time, especially if you live far from the hospital or if you are home alone and would feel more secure in a hospital environment.

Don't panic. Remember that first-time mothers usually take longer to deliver. Please don't think of driving yourself alone! And, if the contractions are very frequent, don't waste time trying to find your doctor. They can call him from the hospital as soon as you get there.

There are three basic signs that will let you know, without a doubt, that the birth has entered the first stage. Any of the following could occur:

Uterine contractions (see discussion above)

With each contraction, the uterus constricts and hardens. The goal of this constricting movement is to stretch the cervix in order to open it enough to allow the baby to exit. After the contraction, it relaxes again. It remains at rest for a fixed length of time until it decides to stretch itself again and produces another contraction.

The final contractions are the most intense, can last up to a whole minute, and can occur every two or three minutes. Usually in this stage, the cervix dilates the necessary amount to allow the baby to exit. Nature in its infinite wisdom manages to have these contractions serve also as a type of stimulating massage for the baby, whose organs and bodily systems are getting ready for the difficult passage into the outside world.

Breaking of the water (rupture of the amniotic membranes)

This refers to the breaking of the superfine membrane containing the amniotic fluid in which the baby has been floating. This fluid's mission has been to protect and keep the fetus warm for nine months. In general, this sac breaks all at once, without causing the mother any pain. However, it can also break and trickle slowly.

The rupture is evident when it is a sudden gush, because about a liter of warm liquid emerges, with a particular odor, wetting your legs. But it can also trickle more slowly, looking similar to the vaginal secretions you have been noticing during the final months of pregnancy.

There is no fixed time for the water to break. It can occur before or during the first contractions, or can be delayed to such a point that the doctor is forced to break it artificially.

Loss of the mucous plug

The cervix has been covered until now by a type of "plug," which is made of mucus and protects the interior of the womb (where the baby is) from the outside world and from any possible contamination. Once dilation begins, this thick layer of mucus, which contains traces of blood (due to the rupturing of several capillaries) comes loose and exits through the vagina, without the mother experiencing any pain.

When this occurs, it signals that the birth is imminent, usually within a few hours. Sometimes, though, days can go by after the mucous plug is lost and before the birth takes place. Or the plug could come loose when the contractions are well established. In any case, it is advisable to tell your doctor when the plug breaks loose.

ARRIVING AT THE HOSPITAL

As soon as you arrive at the hospital with contractions, the doctor or nurse will perform a vaginal exam to determine whether the cervix is dilated, since this is an indication of imminent birth. You will be taken to the predelivery room or to the delivery room if the dilation is very advanced. There is always the possibility that this is a "false alarm," in which case, after your exam, you will be told to go back home until the contractions become longer and occur at more regular intervals.

Rhythmic and painful contractions usually indicate that the cervix has begun to dilate. The cervix has to dilate to ten centimeters (four inches) for the baby to be able to pass through it into the vagina.

As to the duration, intensity, and difficulty of the birth, there is no infallible general rule. It depends on many factors—whether this is your first delivery, how much you have prepared for the delivery, your health, your ability to stand pain and to relax (there are women who experience very little pain), how effective the contractions are, etc.

Usually, if this is a first delivery, labor will be a little longer, lasting on average about fourteen hours from start to finish.

Predelivery or labor room

In the predelivery room, special nurses will prepare you for birth. Depending on the hospital, they will give you an enema, disinfect and wash the genital area, and begin to administer an intravenous solution. Periodically your doctor will give you a pelvic exam to evaluate the degree of dilation of the cervix. Other exams include external and internal monitors to evaluate the contractions and the baby's heartbeat.

There are women who get up, walk, and chat with other mothers-to-be during this period, while others are so uncomfortable, due to the contractions, that they prefer to remain lying down.

You can count on the presence of your husband, family member, or friend in the room with you, depending, of course, on the regulations of your hospital. Therefore, becoming familiar with the procedures of the hospital where you are going to give birth, in order to know what to expect when the time comes, is a good idea.

Final stages of labor

You will notice that the beginning stages of dilation are coming to an end—and that, as a result, your baby's birth is drawing near—when the contractions become more frequent and intense. This final stage is the most painful one. It can last from half an hour up to two hours and, during that time, the contractions can last for one minute at a time and come every two minutes.

The dilation of the cervix is complete when it reaches ten centimeters. It is important that you do everything you can to remain relaxed at the end of this first stage and that you summon the strength to continue. You don't have far to go for those long months of waiting to come to an end! Remember everything you've learned in your relaxation and breathing classes and apply it.

SECOND STAGE OF THE DELIVERY: THE BIRTH

DELIVERY ROOM (ACTIVE PHASE)

When the dilation has reached its peak, you may be moved on a stretcher or gurney to the delivery room. This depends on the hospital; some have labor and delivery in the same room. You will know that you have probably dilated enough when you feel the need to push—although some women may feel the need to push even before they have managed to dilate sufficiently.

Starting now, even though the contractions won't stop, your active participation will allow you to ignore the pain, in a manner of speaking. The final stage of your pregnancy—pushing the baby out—can last for an hour or maybe more for women who have never had children; those who are not first timers already have bodies that are more suited to the task and manage to push the baby out in anywhere from thirty to forty-five minutes, on average.

Pushing and contractions

In the classes you've been attending for several months, they've shown you how to push more effectively so as to make the delivery go faster. Even though it's uncomfortable, there's no special technique required; it's the same pushing that you do when you go to the bathroom—that is, forcing the abdominal muscles. It's *very* important that you know how to combine these pushes with the contractions, which won't stop.

In order to help you coordinate the deep breathing/contraction/pushing process, you will be assisted by qualified personnel who will let you know the exact moment when you should push with all your might. Concentrate on their instructions and do what they tell you when they tell you to do it. This will also help minimize any physical discomfort.

Breathing deeply before each contraction (your body will tell you seconds before it occurs) and holding your breath will allow you to push with more force. You will be encouraged by thinking that the more you push, the quicker the delivery will be. However, always push along with the rhythm of the contractions, taking time to relax and rest between each one.

Also, breathe deeply during those intervals; this will allow your muscles to relax—and you as well—and will enable both your lungs and the baby's to receive more oxygen. In the meantime, the nurse will monitor your baby's heartbeat by means of a special stethoscope.

Remember: **YOU are the heroine of this movie.** Even though your doctor has played a large role up until now, and, following the birth, the baby will steal the show—at the moment of birth, you are the undisputed star. The doctor and the nurse, or the midwife, will indicate when you should push. Your husband can help you with moral support and help remind you to breathe during those moments. But the one who needs to push, with all her might, is you.

PUSHING POSITIONS DURING DELIVERY

- Squatting
- Sitting (i.e., propped up with a cushion or on a special chair)
- Standing
- Lying on your side
- Lying flat on your back with legs extended (this may be the least efficient of all)

The baby's arrival

While you are pushing during the last contractions, deep inside its body the baby will know that the big moment is here. He or she is all rolled up into a ball, with his or her extremities folded inward up against the chest and the wall of the uterus, and his or her little head slightly bending forward.

The baby will adapt to the rhythm of the contractions and the maternal pushing that have opened the birth canal (the vagina), which is sufficiently dilated to accommodate the head. Even though there really isn't a lot of room, the baby will manage.

The baby will make a series of adjusting movements within the womb, which will help sort out the difficulties of passing through the narrow canal. First, he or she places the head at an oblique angle, and then instinctively straightens it out immediately prior to exiting. At that point—this is when the doctor can see your baby's head for the first time—the entire area between the vaginal and anal regions has stretched to its maximum.

The doctor's expert hand will reach out and delicately take the baby's head, moving it slowly so that it moves out more easily. It's possible that, by now, your strength is spent, which is why the medical personnel might help the baby come out by pushing on the base of your uterus.

It used to be common practice—even if the mother had dilated in a satisfactory manner—for the doctor to make a small incision, called an episiotomy, in the vulva. This was done following the application of a local anesthetic. The incision allowed the baby's head to come out more easily and sometimes shortened labor slightly. But several studies published since 2000 show that the episiotomy increased the risk of skin tears and of problems with fecal incontinence after delivery. That is why most doctors today will only perform an episiotomy if the baby appears to be in distress, if the mother is overly exhausted, or if she is in too much pain. It would be wise for you to talk to your doctor about this before your delivery during one of your routine office visits.

Once the head has emerged, it will be much easier for the rest of the baby to come out, with the doctor still assisting by lightly rotating the baby's body in order to place the shoulders parallel to the vulvar opening. This creates a larger space in order to speed the exiting process.

> ## MYTH: IT'S BAD LUCK TO BUY THINGS
> ## FOR THE BABY BEFORE IT IS BORN
>
> Obviously, this is a superstition dating from the time when pregnancy and birth were much more dangerous. Some religious groups still adhere to this notion. There is no scientific basis for it, so use your common sense.

The first minutes

A cry will signal that the baby is breathing on its own for the first time. That is why the mother, the father, and everyone present will be overjoyed to hear the baby's first cry.

Following this, the umbilical cord will be severed and suction will be used to extract any liquid or mucus from the mouth and nose of the newborn. The baby is washed and placed in the arms of her mother.

Once the baby has exited, the contractions cease, except for one last, less painful one, which follows several minutes later, in order to expel the placenta and the rest of the amniotic sac. If necessary the doctor will remove any remaining parts of the placenta that have stayed inside the uterus, in order to prevent subsequent hemorrhaging. Any remaining blood is also expelled from the uterus. After that, the mother is subjected to another series of procedures:

- She receives an injection that stimulates the contraction of the uterus in order to prevent hemorrhaging.
- The episiotomy is stitched together (if an incision was made).
- The pubic and anal areas are washed and disinfected.
- Her pulse, blood pressure, and temperature are taken.
- The medical staff continues to monitor her for a while to ensure that everything is stable, after which she is moved to her room.

METHODS OF DELIVERY

Delivery with anesthesia

There are different types of anesthesia. You should discuss them with your doctor during your office visits. Even though you can never guarantee what you might decide at the time of the delivery, if you feel a great deal of pain you can request anesthesia. It is important that you understand the risks and advantages of anesthesia and that your doctor is well aware of your preferences.

PAIN-RELIEVING MEDICATIONS FALL INTO TWO CATEGORIES

- Analgesics. They relieve pain without causing total loss of sensation. The person is not unconscious while receiving analgesics.
- Anesthetics. They cause total loss of sensation. They can be local anesthetics (removing the pain from specific areas of the body while the patient remains awake) or general anesthetics (causing loss of consciousness).

Analgesics

Analgesics include medications like Meperidine (known as Demerol), which can be given intravenously or intramuscularly (a shot in the buttock). Some women may experience nausea, vomiting, depression, or a mild drop in blood pressure. There is a medication that can be given to counteract these side effects. Depending on the dose and the time when it is given, occasionally the baby may be sleepy at birth.

Anesthetics

There are two main types of *anesthetics:* regional nerve blocks and general anesthesia.

Regional nerve blocks cause a loss of sensation in the area of the nerve (or nerves) that are injected. The advantage is that the woman is awake throughout the whole process. The disadvantage is that nerve blocks may cause delayed labor or may decrease the urge to push during a vaginal delivery.

There are three main types of regional nerve blocks: pudendal, epidural, and spinal.

- *Pudendal Block:* Used shortly before delivery as an injection into the perineal or vaginal area. It is especially useful when forceps are used or to do and/or repair an episiotomy. It does not totally eliminate pain, but it can be helpful, and any complications, should they arise, are minimal.

- *Epidural Block:* It causes loss of feeling below the waist without paralyzing the legs. The anesthetic (i.e., Lidocaine) is given on an as-needed basis through a fine tube, which has been inserted through a needle in the back during labor and delivery. It is given in a space between the bone and the spinal cord, which is protected by the vertebrae that form the spine. Advantages include the ability to increase, decrease, or stop the block, depending on the pain and the stage of labor. It also leaves the mother conscious during the whole process, enabling her to push and actively participate. Among its disadvantages, it can cause a drop in blood pressure in the mother and of the heartbeat in the baby.

- *Spinal Block:* A variation of the epidural block, it causes loss of feeling in the area of the pelvis only. Unlike the epidural, the spinal is injected as a single dose just prior to delivery. It goes into the fluid that surrounds the spinal cord. It is shorter-acting, and side effects are seen less frequently. This is used when forceps are required to deliver the baby.

General anesthesia produces loss of consciousness. It was in widespread use many years ago. Nowadays, it is avoided unless an emergency cesarean must be performed, in cases of hemorrhage, or in cases of breech birth, where the baby is in a seated position instead of facing head down. General anesthesia requires intubation. It is generally avoided due to the risk of complications for the mother as well as the baby. The main disadvantage for the baby is that he or she is sedated at birth. A rare, but serious, complication of this anesthesia in the mother is possible aspiration of food or acid from the stomach to the lungs (causing aspiration pneumonia). Obviously, the possibility of complications is greatly reduced in the hands of qualified professionals.

Cesarean section

This operation, which used to be quite risky and was done only in extreme cases, is now much safer than it used to be, for the baby as well as for the mother. Modern techniques include a transversal incision in the lower and most delicate part of the uterus, and antibiotics have facilitated the recovery as well as minimized complications.

Cesarean sections are required in situations when the birth is not progressing as it should. Some of these are:

- The baby is too large to exit through the mother's birth canal.
- The uterine contractions are not enough to advance the exit of the baby, in spite of the intravenous use of oxytocin. Oxytocin is a hormone normally produced by the body for this purpose.
- The baby is in an abnormal position that doesn't allow it to exit through the vaginal canal. Ideally (and in the vast majority of cases), children are born with their extremities up against their torso and the wall of the uterus and with the head bent down in front and pointing toward the vaginal canal. But it is possible for a baby to be in an abnormal position. For example, in a horizontal position, or seated, either on the buttocks, or the legs. In these cases, there is a risk of the umbilical cord exiting before the baby, which would place the baby's life in danger.
- There is an abnormality in the mother's uterus or the vagina that obstructs the passageway, preventing the baby's exit.
- The mother develops preeclampsia or eclampsia.
- There are abnormalities in the placenta. For example, if there is anything found in or around the cervical area (known as placenta previa, which can bleed before the baby exits), or in cases when the placenta breaks loose before the baby is born (premature detachment of the placenta).
- The mother has a vaginal infection caused by an outbreak of herpes at the time of birth, which could be passed on to the baby if there is a vaginal birth, or if she has uncontrolled diabetes, or if she has a problem with her platelets (which relate to coagulation of the blood).
- Two weeks have passed following the estimated date of delivery, and there is evidence of fetal suffering.
- In certain circumstances when the mother has had previous cesarean sections, the doctor recommends another be performed. Having had a prior cesarean section is not an automatic indication to do another cesarean section, however.

Cesarean sections are not always performed on an emergency basis. Sometimes, depending on the reason for the procedure, the date can be determined beforehand. Whenever possible, it is done between the thirty-sixth and the fortieth weeks of pregnancy, in order to give the baby the maximum time possible to develop and mature inside the uterus.

If a cesarean section is elected, the mother can have it performed under general anesthesia, or she may choose to get an epidural. Emergency cesareans are normally performed under general anesthesia.

Even though recovery from a vaginal birth is quicker and easier than that following a cesarean section, you shouldn't be concerned about the scar. It will be invisible, even when you wear a bikini. The incision is made immediately above, and parallel to, the pubic area. Frequently the incision is covered over once the hair in this area grows back.

If your husband wants to be present for the birth of his baby, a cesarean section is no reason for him not to do so. Many hospitals allow the father to be present during the operation and even prepare him beforehand with special classes so that he isn't shocked by what he sees.

In spite of the fact that a cesarean section is surgery, your recovery is relatively easy and won't prevent you from breast-feeding your baby. Normally, the intravenous solution is removed the next day and you can start to breast-feed within twenty-four hours, even if your stay at the hospital lasts two or three days longer.

Induced delivery

This refers to the stimulation or inducement of the beginning stages of labor, by rupturing the membranes of the amniotic sac (breaking the water) and/or by giving oxytocin intravenously. This hormone is normally produced by the body in larger amounts when the pregnancy reaches its term, in order to allow the uterus to contract.

If more than two weeks have passed beyond your estimated delivery date, or if your water has broken, or if you show other problems (like preeclampsia, etc.), or if there is evidence that the fetus is suffering, your doctor may decide to induce labor and delivery. In these cases, if steps are not taken to speed up the birth, your baby's life and/or your own could be endangered.

There are circumstances in which the birth is induced for the convenience of the mother and/or the doctor. The medical community in general does not endorse this last option.

Delivery using forceps or vacuum extraction

Sometimes the baby's head "gets stuck" during the birth process and does not continue to descend in a normal manner. If this occurs when the baby is high in the birth canal, a cesarean will be performed. But if it occurs when the baby has progressed lower into the canal, the doctor might use forceps or a vacuum extractor to assist with the birth. A forceps is a surgical device resembling large spoons (similar to salad tongs) that is placed around the baby's head in order to extract it gently, after which the body exits in a normal manner. Vacuum extraction uses a plastic cup that is attached to the baby's head and gently pulls the baby through the birth canal by suction. This is the method of choice in Europe.

Some women are afraid of forceps because they've heard stories about babies who suffered complications or deformities resulting from their use. Years ago, forceps were used when the baby had not yet descended low enough in the birth canal. In those cases, the baby had to be pulled with considerable force, a procedure that could, in some cases, cause brain injuries in the fetus.

However, in professional hands, if there is complete dilation of the cervix and if the head is clearly visible (no more than two inches from the vagina), the baby is in no danger whatsoever. The mother can help the doctor as well, avoiding complications by ceasing to push while he or she manipulates the forceps or the vacuum extractor.

LONGEST DELIVERY IN HISTORY

The longest delivery known took place in Rome, Italy. It involved twins. Mrs. Danny Petrungaro gave birth naturally to her daughter Diana on December 22, 1987, and to Monica, Diana's twin sister, thirty-six days later—via cesarean section.

PROBLEMS DURING DELIVERY

Uterine lacerations

Laceration of the cervix occurs occasionally during birth, and when it does, the doctor becomes aware of it immediately. A characteristic symptom of this is excessive bleeding. Once the damage extends beyond two centimeters, the laceration is sutured. The doctor applies an anesthetic before putting in the stitches, if he has not already done so at the beginning of the birth process.

Fetal distress

This complication arises when the fetus does not receive enough oxygen. Causes include:

- Maternal illnesses such as anemia, hypertension, and heart trouble
- Low blood pressure of the mother
- Insufficiency, degeneration, or premature detachment of the placenta
- Compression of the umbilical cord
- Prolonged uterine activity
- Fetal infection

Generally speaking, when there is fetal distress, the mother notices a decrease or total absence of the baby's movement, and the doctor notices changes in the fetus's heartbeat, by listening with a stethoscope or using a special monitor. In each case, the doctor will decide if it is necessary to perform an emergency cesarean section or to perform some other kind of intervention.

Uterine rupture

This complication is rare but dangerous. It generally arises in women who have had incisions in their wombs due to prior cesarean sections or operations for the removal of uterine fibromas. Women who have had four or five children are more prone to suffering this complication, due to the fact that their uterus is more distended. This is a medical emergency.

The symptoms of uterine rupture may include severe abdominal pain, fainting, fast pulse rate, gasping for air, and agitation. Vaginal bleeding does not necessarily have to occur.

Once uterine rupture is identified, it is necessary to take the mother to the operating room immediately and remove the baby. In cases where the rupture is small, the wound can sometimes be repaired with sutures. In severe cases, it is necessary to remove the uterus. There is a high risk of complications, including death, for both mother and baby.

THIRD STAGE OF THE DELIVERY

DELIVERY OF THE PLACENTA

This follows the baby's delivery and usually occurs between five and thirty minutes after detaching from the uterus. If it does not detach completely, the doctor will remove it to avoid subsequent bleeding or infections.

POSTPARTUM PROBLEMS

Even though you may notice certain discomfort in the days following the delivery (see Chapter 12)—such as pain in the area where the episiotomy was performed; pain in the lower part of the abdomen due to uterine contractions; discomfort due to hemorrhoids, constipation, and distended breasts—this is normal. However, you should call your doctor if you experience any of the following symptoms:

- Excessive bleeding that requires the use of more than one sanitary pad every hour over several hours, or if the amount exceeds that of a regular menstrual period, especially after the third or fourth day
- Fever above 100.4 degrees Fahrenheit (or 39 degrees Centigrade) twenty-four hours after giving birth
- Nausea and vomiting
- Burning or an urgent desire to urinate
- Pain or swelling in either or both legs, or pain in one or both calves upon flexing the feet upward
- Pain in your chest, coughing, or shortness of breath
- Reddening or pain confined to one or both breasts
- Persistence or increase in pain in the vagina or anus
- Increase in the amount of vaginal discharge, accompanied by a foul odor
- Pain in the lower part of the abdomen that increases as the days go on and/or secretion from the scar from a cesarean section
- Depression that prevents you from taking care of the baby or coping with daily activities

POSTPARTUM HEMORRHAGE

This could be a serious complication, and it occurs with relative frequency. The main causes include:

- Uterus that is too relaxed and can't contract due to a prolonged labor
- A traumatic delivery
- A very distended uterus due to having had many children
- An exceptionally large fetus or excessive amniotic fluid
- A malformed placenta or a placenta that separated prematurely
- A rupture in the uterus
- Fibromas or tumors that block the uterine contractions
- A deficiency of vitamin K in the mother
- A problem with coagulation in the mother—a low platelet count, for example

Excessive bleeding immediately following the delivery may also occur due to lacerations of the uterus or the vagina that haven't healed. If these occur around a week later, they might be caused by fragments of the placenta that remain in the uterus. In this last case, the mother also suffers pain in the lower part of the abdomen.

The doctor will determine the treatment depending on the cause of the bleeding, which may consist of:

- Massages or medicines like oxytocin and prostaglandin to stimulate contraction of the uterus
- Locating and repairing lacerations
- Removing the fragments of the placenta that remain inside the uterine cavity

Normally, following one of these treatments, the mother will recover with relative ease.

THE FIRST MOMENTS WITH YOUR BABY

It's quite possible that, even before the doctor has cut the umbilical cord, you may want to have contact with your baby's little body. This is possible if the baby is placed on your abdomen, well covered so that he or she doesn't get cold. The difference in temperature between the "cold" environment of the delivery room and the "cozy" environment inside Mom's body where he or she has been growing for nine months is significant.

When the doctor is about to sever the umbilical cord that connects the baby to the placenta, he will ask you to breathe deeply and slowly. At that moment, for the last time, you will be giving your baby the oxygen needed to live. Once separated from the umbilical cord, your baby will undergo a routine performed on all newborns by the hospital medical personnel:

- They apply an antibiotic to his eyes to prevent any infection he might have acquired in the birth canal.
- They remove all traces of amniotic fluid from the respiratory tract.
- They take his pulse and blood pressure.
- They examine his lungs to find out if his breathing is okay.
- They inject vitamin K to facilitate coagulation.
- They do a blood test to determine his blood type and see if he's anemic or has low blood sugar—something that is quite common in babies who are underweight.

Your newborn's condition will be evaluated with the Apgar index. The Apgar measures five characteristics: heartbeat, respiration, muscle tone, reflexes (two kinds), and skin color. Scoring is on a scale from 0 to 10, with 10 being perfect. If your baby gets a rating of 7 or higher, he has been born in good physical shape.

If you suffer from diabetes, or if a problem is suspected arising from the delivery or the examination of the baby, other tests will be done.

If you had planned on breast-feeding your baby, you can take advantage of the moments following the birth to do this for the first time. You will see that your baby will put his lips up to the nipple and will start to suck in an instinctive and natural way. This process stimulates the uterus to return to its normal size and all the organs to move back to the positions they occupied before the pregnancy. Your postpartum recovery period will be shortened the earlier you start to breast-feed your baby; it will also help to increase the production of milk in your breasts.

Don't hesitate to hug and caress your baby as soon as you have him or her in your arms. Remember that the baby not only knows you by your heartbeat but also by your voice. Don't be surprised if he or she follows you attentively from the moment of birth. You will notice that, no matter in which position you hold him or her, the baby will fold his or her arms and legs and adopt a position similar to the one maintained in the womb. This initial contact between you and your baby is crucial to your future relationship.

Following the delivery, in addition to the excitement, you will probably feel exhausted. But don't worry, because nature has already thought of this. Soon you will notice that your baby spends most of his or her time sleeping and wakes up only to eat. And while the baby sleeps, you can really rest . . . for the first time in nine months. Congratulations on your new son or daughter!

STEPHANIE SALAS
Actress and rock singer

I had Michelle—who, as everyone knows, is Luis Miguel's daughter—when I was nineteen. Contrary to what many may think, I took the news that I was pregnant not only very calmly, but with great expectations. This, due to the fact that I understood I was responsible for my actions, allowed me not to be very affected by what my family, people generally, or the press would say. The fact that my mother, Silvia Pasquel, said she would support whatever I decided made me feel very calm during my pregnancy.

I discovered I was pregnant after I went to the doctor to deal with what I thought were parasites that were causing me dizziness and nausea. "What if," I thought to myself, "it turns out that I'm pregnant? No, I'd better go to a gynecologist," I said to myself; "that way I'll feel safer." And sure enough, I was pregnant!

The secret for having had a relatively uncomplicated pregnancy is that I took very good care of myself; I ate very well and also avoided consuming alcohol and smoking. All that, plus the fact that desserts are my weakest point. I tried not to indulge. If I felt I had passed the limit, I would eliminate bread and tortillas from my meals and have a light dinner. I recommend that pregnant women never stop exercising.

Since it is common that when you're very young and get pregnant you will develop acne or pimples on your face, I solved the problem by seeing a cosmetologist, who recommended using a cream. Now, more because of my desire to have a healthy and beautiful complexion, I apply mud or nopal juice masks.

Chapter 12

FINAL CONSIDERATIONS

WHAT YOUR NEW BABY LOOKS LIKE

- Don't be scared if your baby's head seems too large in relation to the rest of his or her body (at birth, the head is one-quarter the size of the body). This is natural, and in time, it will look more normal. Babies delivered vaginally occasionally have a slightly "pointed" head, or they might have a slight inflammation and a violet coloring on their heads, but this is temporary. If it was a breech birth, there will be a slight inflammation and violet coloring on the buttocks, but it is also temporary.
- Sometimes the newborn's ears seem large and/or stick out too far. After a few months, they too will look more normal. Naturally, when you lay your baby on his side, make sure that the ear isn't folded over.
- Even if your baby is born with more hair than Gloria Trevi, that mane will fall out during the first six months and will be followed by hair that might be totally different in terms of texture and color.
- You will notice hair covering parts of the newborn's face and body. Don't worry, this will fall out in due course.

- Infants, especially those born after forty weeks, can have extra long nails; you should trim the nails so that the baby won't scratch himself or herself by accident.
- The obvious irritation in newborns' eyes (caused by the drops placed in the eyes at birth) will disappear in less than three days, as will the accompanying inflammation. If you notice a secretion from the eyes, especially seventy-two hours or more after birth, notify your doctor.
- Infants' eyes also seem to be squinting, but this is due to the deep creases at the base of the eyes—which will disappear in time. During these first few days or weeks, the baby's eyes—not having very strong muscles yet—tend to look crossed. This is perfectly normal in the newborn, but if this condition persists by the time he or she is six months old, you should see a doctor.
- Don't think that, because the baby looks like you when born, he or she is going to become your spitting image. Newborns change a lot during the first few months, and by New Year's, he could end up looking a lot more like his grandfather than his father!

YOUR FIGURE FOLLOWING DELIVERY

A study conducted by the University of Alabama showed that women who give birth are more prone to being overweight and to having a wider waistline than those who don't have children. However, the study—which took five years and involved some 1,200 women between the ages of eighteen and thirty—also showed that not having children was no guarantee for maintaining a slender figure.

Results showed that African American women who didn't have children have a greater chance of gaining twice as much weight as childless white women. White women who had their first child during the study retained around ten extra pounds, but they retained only seven pounds after the second birth. African American women who had children during the study retained some twenty pounds after the first pregnancy, and eleven after the second.

The good news is that Hispanic men tend to like us "a little on the plump side."

POSTPARTUM DISCOMFORTS

PHYSICAL

There are several physical discomforts that can arise during the days following the delivery. The following are the most common:

Body aches

These are due to all the effort required during labor and delivery. It's as if you'd just run a marathon.

Abdominal (belly) pain

The cramps you feel in your abdomen—especially when you're breast-feeding the baby—which last several days, indicate that your uterus is going back to its normal size, since it was distended at the time of delivery. Don't worry, this is normal. If you find it very uncomfortable, your doctor can recommend an analgesic (a pain medicine that will not affect the baby even though you're breast-feeding). If you had a cesarean section, pain is probably localized in the incision that is healing, and there may also be a slight swelling due to gas. Walking and drinking lots of fluids can help move the bowels and get rid of the gas.

Pain at the stitches

With vaginal birth, the majority of internal stitches dissolve within a week, and the external ones will fall out of their own accord; until that occurs, indicating that your wound has healed, they may be uncomfortable. You can speed up the healing process by doing pelvic exercises on the floor—like the ones you did prior to the birth—as soon as you feel better.

It's also important to keep these areas clean at all times. Take a warm bath and dry the area well without pulling on them. If the stitches hurt a lot, place a bag of ice, wrapped in a towel, over them.

In the case of external stitches or clamps used in cesarean sections, they will be removed by your doctor in about seven days.

Excessive urination

It is normal to urinate frequently during the first days following the birth, since your body is eliminating excess fluid. Upon urinating, you might feel slight discomfort; that area is extremely sensitive right now. Nevertheless, if you drink lots of fluids, your urine will be less concentrated and will cause you less discomfort.

Vaginal bleeding

It's normal to experience vaginal bleeding for two to six weeks after the delivery. Women who breast-feed stop bleeding faster. In the beginning, the blood is a deep red, but after three or four days, it turns brown.

It's possible for this bleeding to last until your first postpartum menstrual period. During this time, you should use sanitary pads instead of tampons (the latter can increase the risk of infection).

Constipation

Constipation is very common for twenty-four to forty-eight hours after the delivery. Walking stimulates bowel movement, as does drinking lots of water and juices and eating high-fiber foods (such as fruit, vegetables, cereal, etc.). Try not to force it too much. If you have stitches, it would be highly unlikely that they would rupture with the effort of having a bowel movement. However, if you feel more comfortable, you can press lightly on the area with the stitches, using a clean sanitary pad, when you want to have a bowel movement.

Excessive perspiration

If you notice excessive perspiration during the week following the delivery, especially at night, don't worry. This could be due to hormonal changes and the elimination of fluids retained during the pregnancy. If you think you have a fever, take your temperature. If your thermometer registers 100.4 Fahrenheit (38 Celsius) or more after twenty-four hours, call your doctor.

Hemorrhoids

Some women experience discomfort due to postpartum hemorrhoids. These are veins that swelled as a result of the increased pressure in the pelvic area when you were pushing during the delivery. The ones that swell up as a result of the birthing effort disappear two or three days later.

Unfortunately, if the hemorrhoids appeared during the course of the pregnancy, they could bother you for several months. The ice packs I mentioned for the stitches, warm sitz baths, and several creams and locally applied suppositories (your doctor can recommend some) will help. Avoid constipation as much as possible.

Swollen breasts

Your breasts will not show much change in the first three days following the delivery, except for the presence of colostrum, the yellowish liquid that is a precursor to breast milk. However, they will become swollen on the third or fourth day and will feel warm and become engorged with veins, causing a sharp pain that could reach from your armpits to your back.

This painful sensation won't go away until your baby establishes his or her feeding cycle, if, indeed, you have decided to breast-feed. If, on the other hand, you decide to bottle-feed, you will find relief by wearing a tight brassiere and by using ice packs and analgesics (pain medicines) until the medicine that the doctor gave you to stop milk production takes effect. In this case, do not, under any circumstances, extract milk. This would stimulate your mammary glands and cause your breasts to get full again.

Hair loss

There are times in your life that could cause you to lose your hair, such as periods of severe nervous tension or crash diets. But perhaps the most surprising hair loss occurs following birth. During the pregnancy, and right through the birth, a series of factors affect the female body and the hair. The increase of certain hormones during the pregnancy, in many cases, makes the hair maintain its normal state, or even improve.

But, in the postpartum period, the decrease in hormones—along with the decrease of certain minerals—might make you lose a lot of hair during the next three- to six-month period (sometimes you don't notice this until you stop breast-feeding). Don't buy a wig yet! The hair will grow back. Just maintain a balanced diet and keep taking your vitamin and mineral supplements for a couple of months. Once the breast-feeding period is over and your menstrual cycles have resumed their normal rhythm, you'll notice continued recovery and your hair will grow back the same as before.

IT'S NOT ONLY NINE MONTHS

A study undertaken by researchers at the University of Minnesota proved that traditional ideas that a woman only needs six weeks to recover from a vaginal birth—and eight weeks to recover from a cesarean section—may be mistaken. According to the study, one month after birth many women were still complaining of discomfort in their breasts, lack of appetite, fatigue, and hot flashes.

Many of these problems persisted three months after the delivery, and 40 percent of the new mothers complained of pain during sex. Nine months after giving birth, many of them continued to have vaginal discomfort and constipation. Twenty percent of the new mothers in this study suffered from discomfort during sex a full year after giving birth. If you experience continuing discomfort, talk to your doctor.

EMOTIONAL PROBLEMS

Postpartum depression

You just came home from the hospital with your baby in your arms. Finally, after nine months of concern and anxiety, you have with you this being whom you love more than anything or anyone in the world. The baby's room has everything that's needed to be comfortable. Your husband or partner seems to be the happiest man on earth, and he can't do enough to please you and to help you change diapers, take care of the baby, etc. What more can you ask from life?

However . . . you feel a sense of unbearable emptiness, which often makes you cry for no reason. You're not sick. You're experiencing a phenomenon that—even though science is not exactly sure why—we know occurs to a lot of women after giving birth. It is known as postpartum depression, or postpartum "blues."

There are several theories regarding its cause. Some experts think it is due to the fact that, when the mother gives birth, she is physically separated from the baby she carried inside herself for so many months. Now the baby ceases to be totally dependent on her for food and oxygen. Now he or she is a person, whom the mother has to grow to love and to get used to.

On the other hand, the attention that the family gave the pregnant woman before the birth now drifts toward the child. These considerations are coupled with new responsibilities that the new mother has to get used to: taking care of the baby day and night, without neglecting her household duties.

In addition, the fatigue and the hormonal changes the body of the new mother undergoes make her feel extremely sensitive, overreacting at certain moments and causing her to be melancholic and sad. This can last for several weeks following the birth of the baby.

THE DEPRESSION STARTS EARLIER

In two out of three women who suffer from postpartum depression, the symptoms start during the last months of pregnancy. According to a study presented at a symposium in Geneva, loneliness is the chief cause of prepartum depression, which is usually accompanied by anxiety, physical problems, and insomnia. According to the researchers, psychotherapy should begin with the first symptoms, before the delivery, in order to achieve the most satisfactory results.

How to overcome it

In order to combat this state, you have to accept the fact that you're not "superwoman," and you should allow others to help you take care of the baby and the housework, especially at the beginning, until you start adjusting to your new routine.

Personal appearance plays an important role in how new mothers feel. Forget about those extra pounds, which you will lose little by little, and recover your feminine charm. Take a shower, put on perfume, and look pretty when your husband comes home. Having just given birth doesn't mean you are ill, so stop wearing nightgowns and robes all day— they only make you feel worse.

Visit and share with other women who've gone through the same experience, and try to learn from them. And sometimes, after feeding your baby, leave him with someone you trust and go out for a walk with your husband, or go out to eat at a place you both like. That will help you feel less like a diaper-changing machine, and you will prove to yourself that you are still as attractive to your husband as before.

There are severe cases in which depression prevents a woman from carrying out the most mundane everyday tasks—even taking care of the baby—or situations that persist for more than a couple of weeks. In these cases, notify your doctor. This is important. There are treatments that can help you. This situation does not indicate weakness of character. No matter what everyone around you says, if you have any doubts, talk to your doctor.

THE RETURN OF BREAST-FEEDING

After years of using formula for babies, doctors report that breast-feeding is on the rise again. A study performed in 1994 showed that 56 percent of new mothers are breast-feeding their babies, and 19 percent are still breast-feeding six months after the birth. Studies have shown that babies who breast-feed have fewer ear infections, fewer allergies, fewer problems with diarrhea, and that their mothers have a smaller chance of contracting breast cancer.

ADVANTAGES OF BREAST-FEEDING

Biologically speaking, with certain exceptions (women with certain diseases), every woman is prepared to breast-feed her baby. Unfortunately, not everyone can. Sometimes there are practical considerations—for example, some women have to go back to work after six or eight weeks, they're gone for the better part of the day, and they can't deal with breast pumps. Others prefer not to breast-feed because they feel more comfortable with bottle-feeding. A small number of women decide not to breast-feed for aesthetic reasons. They think it will change the shape of their breasts. Don't feel guilty if you cannot breast-feed. The decision to breast-feed is a very personal one, which every woman must make. If you have doubts about breast-feeding, or think you have a condition that would prevent breast-feeding, don't hesitate to ask all the necessary questions in order to get the answers. Even women who have inverted nipples can breast-feed.

I suggest that, if you can, you breast-feed your baby. There is no artificial formula that surpasses the benefits of mother's milk. Among other things, mother's milk changes composition according to the development and needs of the infant. It's better, not just because of its nutritive content, but because nature wisely allows certain antibodies from the mother to get into the milk to protect the baby from specific infections, while he or she is unable to do so himself or herself.

As to its composition, colostrum—which is the initial secretion from the breasts immediately following the birth—is made up of water, proteins, minerals, and elements the newborn needs for nourishment and to be able to expel the meconium (the fecal matter that has been accumulating in his or her intestines during pregnancy).

Throughout the next several days, the breast milk contains larger amounts of proteins, fats, and other substances, which are necessary for the normal development of your baby.

The amount of milk produced during the first few days may be rather sparse, which will cause the baby to cry and require constant feeding. Don't despair and give up—the more the baby sucks, the more prolactin will be secreted. Prolactin is a hormone that stimulates the production of milk in your body. In a couple of days, the baby will ask to be fed every three or four hours and will be quite satisfied. You will know that the baby is full because he or she will be calm and will gain weight as expected.

There are numerous studies that indicate that babies who have been breast-fed grow up to be much healthier than those who were bottle fed. Mother's milk contains—in addition to the antibodies I mentioned, which protect him or her from contracting certain infections—substances that protect him or her from allergies, as well as enzymes that aid in digestion.

Other benefits of breast-feeding include:

- Assisting the uterus to contract and, therefore, allowing other organs to return to the place they occupied prior to your pregnancy
- Establishing a more intimate bond between you and your child, which will help your child to feel protected and safe
- Not having to worry about sterilizing bottles, regulating the temperature of the milk, or measuring the amount. No refrigeration is needed because it never goes bad. Besides, you don't have to stick to a schedule, and you will save money on the cost of baby formula.

LEARNING TO BREAST-FEED

Even though breast-feeding your baby is a natural process, you definitely have to learn how, as with everything else in life. Following are some suggestions that will make it easier and more efficient:

- Wash your nipples with water only. Don't use soap, alcohol, premedicated towelettes, or any disinfectant. Careful cleansing, and keeping them dry, will prevent irritation.

- Try to sit in a comfortable position, preferably one that allows you to support the arm that is holding the baby. You can use a pillow for this if you wish. Relax your shoulders so that you won't get tired as quickly.

- Hold the baby with head higher than stomach, so that he or she won't fill up with gas. With your free hand, use the index fingers and your thumb to hold the breast and make the nipple emerge, or hold the nipple like a cigarette. Leave some room so that the baby can suck on the areola as well. If he or she grabs hold of only the nipple, this will not put pressure on the glands that contain the milk and might cause the nipple to crack and/or hurt. The first few times, the baby will probably get tired right away and go to sleep. But you can wake up the baby by patting him or her gently on the cheeks so that he or she continues to suck. You will know he or she is sucking if you see rhythmic movement of the cheeks.

- Sometimes the baby will stop sucking because your breast is covering the nose and the baby can't breathe well. If this is the case, push your breast slightly in the area just above her or his face so that you uncover the nose.

- If the baby stops feeding but still has the nipple in his or her mouth, slide your finger over the breast and gently insert it between his or her lips at the corner of the mouth. This will allow air to enter and prevent the nipple from being hurt by being let go all at once.

- Upon finishing, place the baby on your shoulder, or facedown on your thighs, and pat the back gently so as to stimulate a burp to expel any gas.

- Never breast-feed from just one side. Start with five minutes on each side and, little by little, increase the time until you reach ten minutes on each side. This is what the baby usually needs to empty each breast completely.

- If at the beginning, the baby can't empty the breasts, try to extract the remaining milk yourself, in order to prevent obstructions in your breasts. Obstructions occur when there is milk residue in the breast ducts; they cause swelling and hardening of the breast—which prevents your baby from latching on in order to suck—and are very painful. In severe cases, infection can occur. If you feel feverish and/or you notice an area of the breast turning red, painful, and hot, call your doctor.

- If you need or want to go out without the baby, or you're very tired, don't worry. You can extract milk with a pump, which is sold at any pharmacy, transfer it into a sterilized bottle, and keep it in the refrigerator until feeding time.

DIET DURING BREAST-FEEDING

Basically you should continue the same balanced diet you maintained during your pregnancy and, if you are below your ideal weight, increase your intake by at least another 500 calories. In addition, don't stop taking the prenatal vitamins and minerals and the calcium supplement that the doctor prescribed for you. And make sure to drink eight glasses of liquids a day (or more, if it's hot).

It is generally recommended that you avoid caffeine, tobacco, alcohol, and drugs, since you can pass these on to the baby through your milk. Remember that certain foods that produce digestive upsets in you might also affect your baby. These might include foods with a lot of onion and garlic, or foods that are cabbage-based. They could also change the taste of your milk, prompting the baby to reject it. If you see that there is a relationship between your consumption of certain foods and your baby eating less and/or having colic or gas, then avoid those foods.

Even though you are eager to regain the figure that you had before the pregnancy, you should lose weight little by little. Weight-loss diets can be harmful to your baby when you're breast-feeding, so be patient and remember that it's worth being a little plump (within limits) for a few more months if this is the price you have to pay to have a healthy baby. Your doctor or a qualified nutritionist can help you determine this.

It's important for you to know that, even though you're breast-feeding and you haven't had your period, you could become pregnant again. If you don't want any surprises, you should take precautions. It's better to use condoms, a diaphragm, etc. But if birth control pills are your choice, the low-dose pills containing only progestins would be best. Although they are less effective than the combined (estrogen or progesterone) pills, their risk of reducing milk output is also decreased. Ask your doctor.

Choose blouses and dresses that button in front. These will facilitate nursing your baby in comfort. You may have to buy larger brassieres, because your bust size will increase considerably. Make sure they fit comfortably, neither too tight nor too loose; bras that open in the front will be very convenient as you will not have to undress each time you nurse.

In time, your baby will go for longer periods between feedings and you will notice that your breasts will leak when it's time for the baby to get hungry. To avoid soiling your clothing, use protective pads in your brassiere, especially when you go out.

BOTTLE-FEEDING

There are a great many kinds of formulas on the market, and your doctor will recommend which one to give your baby. In general, it is advisable to use the kind that is most similar to mother's milk. Formula is sold in two forms: liquid or powder; the latter is prepared by mixing with boiled water.

As opposed to maternal milk, which requires no special preparation and protects the baby against various types of infections, formulas require a series of steps and a great deal of hygiene in their preparation:

- Bottles and containers that are used to mix the formula must be carefully sterilized before using.
- The powder should be stored and covered tightly in its original container, and the liquid formula should be refrigerated.
- The remaining milk not drunk by the baby should be thrown out, so that germs that could cause gastroenteritis (an infection in the digestive tract) don't get inside it.

When preparing the formula, follow the instructions to the letter and never increase or decrease the amount you give your baby without the doctor's orders. He or she is the only one who knows whether the amount is adequate for your baby's size and weight. If your baby develops an allergy to the formula, your doctor will recommend another formula with a soy milk base, instead of cow's milk.

As a matter of fact, there are three types of formula. All are designed to be digested by your baby and fulfill your baby's needs. Most are made out of modified cow's milk. If your doctor determines that your baby doesn't tolerate this type of formula, he or she will recommend a soy-based formula or a formula based on another protein. Regular cow's milk or soy milk cannot be substituted for baby formulas. Symptoms suggestive of an allergy or intolerance to a formula may include abdominal pain, diarrhea, vomiting, and skin rashes. Your doctor will recommend the best formula for your baby. Many formulas have added iron.

It is extremely important that you do not give your baby a bottle while he or she is lying down. He or she could choke, and in the future, when the baby's teeth start coming in, the baby could develop cavities.

Ideally, it is advisable that the bottle containing the formula be warm when given to the baby. Always check the temperature by putting a few drops on the back of your hand before giving it to your infant. When you are giving a bottle to a newborn, hold him or her in your arms. Don't give the baby a bottle while he or she is lying down in the crib, and make sure the baby is swallowing milk, not air. Air can cause gas and colic.

If you feed your baby on a regular schedule from the beginning, every three or four hours, he or she will soon get used to it and will drink until full at each feeding, remaining calm until it's time for the next one.

Even though this sounds simple, with certain babies it isn't. You have to be patient and remember that not all babies are the same, and that some take longer to adapt to a feeding schedule. You will be surprised to learn that some don't feed at night for the first few weeks of life, while others wake up like clockwork every three or four hours for several months.

CHANGING DIAPERS

Newborns may require diaper changes up to ten times a day. It is important to make sure that you have everything you need before you change your baby, including baby wipes to clean him or her with. Those wipes will help remove germs that can cause infections. It's important to always clean your baby from the front to the back. This will avoid introducing bacteria into the urinary tract.

Place the baby in the center of the diaper at waist level. If the navel hasn't dried up, clean it with a little alcohol and place the diaper below it.

The best times to change diapers are:

- Before or after each meal
- After each bowel movement
- Before going to sleep or when baby wakes up
- Before going out
- And, especially, when the baby lets you know that she or he wants to be changed

Keeping the diaper dry helps prevent rashes. To prevent a rash, you can also apply a thin layer of zinc oxide ointment or Vaseline to the diaper area. Removing the diaper for a while during the day will also help keep the area ventilated and decrease the risk of developing diaper rash.

In order for your baby to be more comfortable, select the right diaper size. Disposable diapers have sizes according to the baby's weight.

To keep the baby comfortable while you change him or her, experts recommend that you give the baby a toy—this can be a toy that you give the baby only when you change his or her diaper—or you can make up a song that you sing when you change the baby's diaper.

When it is time for your baby to start using the bathroom, which usually happens between eighteen and thirty months, you can use training pants. Your baby can learn to put them on and take them off like underwear.

BABY'S FIRST VISIT TO THE DOCTOR

You should take your baby to the pediatrician when he or she is two weeks old. The doctor will weigh him or her, but don't be worried if there isn't a marked weight gain. Babies usually lose some weight during the first week. The doctor will also measure the length of the baby and measure the circumference of his or her head and torso.

During this first visit to the doctor, he or she will advise you as to feeding schedules, hours of sleep, colic, changing diapers, etc. Take advantage of this visit to address any questions you have, no matter how silly they may seem.

Find out how often you should take the baby to the doctor, as well as the vaccination program to follow. Usually, the first vaccinations against polio, diphtheria, whooping cough, and tetanus occur at two months.

YOUR RECOVERY PROCESS

The three or four weeks following the birth are known as puerperium. In this stage, your body goes through a series of changes in order to return to its prepregnancy state. The most striking change manifests itself by means of uterine contractions, sometimes painful, which are known as "after pains." If the discomfort is very persistent, you can ask the doctor to prescribe an analgesic (pain medicine).

Good personal hygiene is always important, but even more so while you are experiencing the vaginal bleeding known as *lochia,* which usually lasts around twenty days.

If you are breast-feeding your baby, it's possible that your first menstruation will take some time to return. If you are not breast-feeding, it's very likely that it will return two months after the birth. In both cases, if you want to avoid another pregnancy, it is advisable to use a condom or a diaphragm. Following the first menstruation, an intrauterine device (IUD), a device your doctor places inside the uterus, can be used. Birth control pills are also an option that you should discuss with your doctor. Naturally, in the meantime, you can resume sexual intercourse approximately six weeks after giving birth. This depends on how you feel, whether you had a vaginal delivery or a cesarean, and if the lochia has stopped. To be really sure, check with your doctor.

In order to recover the muscle tone you had before you became pregnant, continue the recommended exercises you did while pregnant, mainly the abdominal and pelvic ones. The doctor will tell you when the best time is to resume your normal exercise routine, but that depends on your lifestyle up until this time, and how fast you have recovered following the delivery—especially if you have had a cesarean.

Recovery following a cesarean will be much faster if you get out of bed as soon as possible and walk around, in order to increase blood flow.

Ideally, you should spend around four months with your baby before going back to work, so that you have enough time to get to know one another and establish a daily routine. If, for any reason, you have to go back to work before this, try to spend as much time as possible with your baby, especially during those first few months.

You will probably feel upset during these first few weeks because you still weigh several pounds more than before the pregnancy. But going on a diet right away could be counterproductive. You will need lots of energy to recover from the delivery and face your new tasks, especially if you are nursing your baby. You will see that, by eating a balanced diet and engaging in a regular exercise program, you will return to your previous size in just a few months.

"If I feel fine after giving birth, do I have to see the doctor after I'm released from the hospital?"

Yes. A doctor's visit is recommended between two to six weeks after delivery. This is to make sure that, if there were any lacerations or if stitches were used, everything has healed. Also, he or she can make sure that the uterus has returned to its normal size following the birth. (This generally occurs at six weeks.)

An orange peel was the first thing used, centuries ago, as a contraceptive diaphragm.

PLANNING YOUR NEXT PREGNANCY

From a health standpoint, it is ideal to wait at least one or two years between pregnancies. When the time comes to plan the birth of your next child, the first thing you and your husband or partner should do is have a medical exam to rule out any medical problems. Then, correct or control any that are detected. You should see your dentist and, besides getting your annual cleaning, have him or her take X-rays (if needed) and fill any cavities you may have. Remember that X-rays are not recommended during pregnancy.

If you still haven't done so, choose an obstetrician whom you want as your doctor. Women who have regular menstrual cycles every twenty-eight days know that their most fertile period is in the middle of the cycle. If they have sexual intercourse during those days, their probability of conceiving is very high. For women with irregular cycles, it's harder to determine the exact day of ovulation. There are several things that can help, for example, taking your temperature on a daily basis. When ovulation occurs, there is a slight rise in temperature (without causing a fever, naturally). There are also some kits that are sold over-the-counter in pharmacies, which—based on a urine sample—can help determine whether you are ovulating.

Obviously, if this is your second child you can be a little more relaxed, knowing that you've already carried a pregnancy to term. If you've had previous abortions or if there are hereditary diseases or congenital malformations in the family or in your first child, your obstetrician could give you some specific recommendations, perform certain tests, or refer you to a geneticist, should that be necessary.

While you are trying to get pregnant, you should avoid exposure to chemical agents and radiation, and—of course—avoid smoking, alcohol, and drugs. Staying away from these will increase your chances of conceiving a healthy baby.

If your first child is preschool age, consider starting him or her in nursery school. It is very likely that he or she will start to feel jealous once his little brother or sister is born. Starting to relate to other children at an early stage will help entertain your first child and prevent him or her from feeling that he or she has been given up, which could occur should you send him or her to school after the "intruder" arrives at home.

Only around 27 percent of the babies born each year were not planned by their parents.

DELIA FIALLO

Writer of *Morelia, Cristal, Maria Elena, Topacio, Esmeralda, Peregrina,* and other well-known "telenovelas"

Each of my five pregnancies and deliveries was different. The first was very normal. The water broke at twelve, and at six I was delivering. The second delivery, I went in without any pain. The doctor said, "Sleep, this will take a while." But when I turned over to go to sleep, I suddenly felt the girl coming out! It turned out that I was already having contractions, but hadn't realized. They barely had time to say, "Keep your legs closed!" and run me to the delivery room. . . .

The day my fourth daughter was born, I had spent the whole day cleaning a huge bookshelf and doing a lot of exercise. I was still fixing up the new house we had just moved into. Typical of the mess involved in moving, when I went to take a bath that night there was no water, no soap, and no electricity! I took my bath by candlelight, with freezing water from a fountain and dishwashing detergent. . . . I don't know if that did it, but that same night I went into labor. It was my only delivery with some complications, because the baby presented itself face forward. However, the doctor managed to straighten her out to a normal position and there was no need for a cesarean section.

After the fourth, I had decided not to have any more children. I was already forty and was avoiding becoming pregnant. But I am an only child and had always said I would have as many children as God sent me. Also, I have always been a staunch enemy of abortion. So, when I became pregnant once more, I never once gave a thought to terminating it; I did, though, ask the doctor for a cesarean section and a tubal ligation. I had already been given an epidural (anesthesia) and was on the table when, within two or three minutes, I heard a baby crying. I thought it must belong to another woman who had just given birth in the same delivery room, when I heard my doctor saying to me, "Male, a boy, masculine!" I had just given birth to my first boy and hadn't even realized it! All this seems to have happened yesterday . . . and yet, all my children are already parents, and I'm a grandmother with twelve grandchildren.

The pregnant woman I most remember from my novelas is Milagros from *A Girl Named Milagros*. The actress, Rebeca Gonzalez, became pregnant halfway through the romance, and I had to make the character also become pregnant. I had to follow that pregnancy, chapter by chapter, as though it were mine! Later, even the baby appeared in the story in the hospital where it was born.

SERVICES THAT ASSIST
THE EXPECTANT MOTHER

I would like to invite you to visit my Web site, www.DoctoraAliza.com, for more information. Please feel free to send any suggestions, comments, or questions. I will also let you know about my upcoming books.

USEFUL TELEPHONE NUMBERS, ADDRESSES, AND WEB SITES

AIM Program/Medical services during pregnancy, (800) 433-2611 (English/Spanish). Mailing address: Access for Infants and Mothers Program, PO Box 15559, Sacramento, CA 95852-0559. www.aim.ca.gov/english/AIMHome.asp. Spanish on Web site.

American Academy of Husband-Coached Childbirth, (800) 4-A-Birth. (English/Spanish). Will answer your questions on natural childbirth (in other words, at home and with the baby's father's help). They will send you a directory listing experts in these methods across the country and a catalog of videos on natural childbirth. You may write to: PO Box 5224, Sherman Oaks, CA 91413. www.bradley.com/. No Spanish on Web site.

American College of Nurse-Midwives, (240) 485-1800. They will locate a professional midwife in your area. Web site: www.midwife.org/. No Spanish on Web site.

A.O.E.C. (Association of Occupational and Environmental Clinics), (202) 347-4976; toll-free (888) 347-AOEC (2632). Evaluation of the pregnant mother's exposure to potential risks at work. They have a network of more than 60 clinics within the United States and, if you call them, they can provide information on the clinics in your area where you can seek help. Address: 1010 Vermont Ave. NW, Suite 513, Washington, DC 20005. Web site: www.aoec.org/ No Spanish on Web site. E-mail: aoec@aoec.org.

A.S.P.O./Lamaze, (800) 368-4404; local: (202) 367-1128 (English/Spanish). Specializes in guidance and offering courses on the Lamaze method. At their toll-free number, they will guide you as to the Lamaze group closest to your area. They also offer the *Lamaze Magazine for Parents,* an English/Spanish publication with useful information on the famous method. You may request it by calling the toll-free number or writing to: 2025 M St. NW, Suite 800, Washington, DC 20036-3309. www.lamaze.org/. No Spanish on Web site.

Association of Birth Defect Children, (407) 895-0802; (800) 313-ABDC (Birth Defect Registry Hotline). Support for families whose babies have been born with defects supposedly produced by the mothers' exposure to drugs, radiation, chemicals, or pesticides. Address: 930 Woodcock Road, Suite 225, Orlando, FL 32803. www.birthdefects.org. No Spanish on Web site.

Breastfeeding.com, Inc. www.breastfeeding.com. No Spanish on Web site. Information and support about the benefits of breast-feeding.

Cesarean Support, Education & Concern, (508) 877-8266. Offers support and information to women who have had or will have a cesarean section delivery. A recording always answers their number, so the best thing is to write to them (and include a self-addressed stamped envelope) at: C.S.E.C., 22 Forest Rd., Framingham, MA 01701. Or you may leave your number after the message and they will call you back collect.

The Confinement Line. Offers support and encouragement to those women who are forced to stay in bed due to dangerous pregnancies. You may write to: PO Box 1609, Springfield, VA 22151.

Depression After Delivery, Inc., (800) 967-7636. Offers support and information to women who suffer "post-partum blues." They have a brochure and 55 groups across the country. If you leave your name and address on their answering service, they will mail you the information. Address: 91 East Somerset St. Raikan, NJ 08869. www.depressionafterdelivery.com/Home.asp. Spanish on Web site.

I Am Your Child Foundation. Information on the importance of the child's brain development from conception to the first years of life. It includes brochures and videos with celebrities that provide parents with insightful tips on how to better care for and protect their child, as well as how to prepare him or her for school and for life. Available in English and in Spanish. Web site: www.iamyourchild.org. In California you may request the new parents kit free of charge, at (800) KIDSO25. (202) 238-4878 (Washington, DC office); (310) 285-2385 (California office).

Infant Formulas by Abbot Laboratories. Similac and others. Web site: www.welcomeaddition.com. English. No Spanish on Web site. (800) 227-5767.

Infant Formulas by Enfamil. Information on nutrition, feeding, pregnancy, and Enfamil. www.enfamil.com.

INFOLINE-MEDICAL also known as 211 LA County, 211 or (800) 339-6993 (English/Spanish). Provides general information and referral to different programs of the Department of Public Social Services, including Medical, Welfare, and many others. www.infoline-la.org/. No Spanish on Web site.

International Childbirth Education Association, Inc., (800) 624-4934; (952) 854-8660. This group is devoted to guiding mothers on their health and the different alternatives for delivery by providing lists of organizations that offer pregnancy classes in different areas. Web site: www.icea.org/. No Spanish on Web site.

Internet Government Pregnancy Resources. Web site: www.healthfinder.gov. English and Spanish.

La Leche League, (800) LALECHE or (800) 525-3243; (847) 519-7730 (The last number provides access to an automated system for finding LLL Leaders in the U.S. by entering a local zip code.). This international organization, started in 1956, supports, educates, and informs mothers who breast-feed their babies. They offer a brochure, schedules for meetings in several cities, and a telephone help line. Write to: PO Box 1209, Franklin Park, IL 60131. Web site: www.lalecheleague.org. Spanish on Web site (www.lalecheleague.org/LangEspanol.html). Spanish materials.

March of Dimes, (800) MODIMES or (888) 663-4637. Information on pregnancy and the prevention of birth defects. Web site: www.modimesmarchofdimes.orgcom. Spanish Web site: www.nacersano.org/.

MEDLINE plus. Pregnancy and reproduction topics. Medical terms, libraries, publications. Web site: www.nlm.nih.gov/medlineplus/pregnancyandreproduction.html. English.

Minnesota Early Learning Design (MELD), (612) 332-7563. Offers mothers information covering the final three months of pregnancy through the third year of the baby's life. There are programs for adolescent mothers, parents with hearing problems, Hispanic families, and parents of invalid children. If you write, they will inform you of centers in your area where these programs are offered. They also have simple books in Spanish about infant care *(New Family, This Book Is for You),* a baby's diary *(New Adventures),* and posters with tables that allow you to follow the baby's development step-by-step. Request their book catalog by calling or writing to: 219 North 2nd St., Suite 200, Minneapolis, MN 55401. Web site: www.meld.org/. No Spanish on Web site. E-mail: info@meld.org.

Mother and Infant Care, www.childbirth.org. Pregnancy, delivery, and child care.

The Mother's Development Center, (800) 645-3828; in New York (516) 529-2929. A support and research system, encompassing 80 national groups, to assist pregnant women and mothers in general.

NAPSAC (National Association of Parents & Professionals for Safe Alternatives in Childbirth), (573) 238-2010. Offers information and support related to delivery at home, the family's care of the mother, and midwife services. At a cost of $7.95 plus $2 shipping and handling (check or money order), they offer a national directory of people who practice alternative delivery methods. Address: NAPSAC Directory, Route 4, Box 646, Marble Hill, MO 63764. Web site: www.napsac.org/. No Spanish on Web site. E-mail: napsac@clas.net.

National AIDS Hotline, (800) CDC-INFO (1-800-232-4636), 24 hours a day, 7 days a week, in English, en español. AIDS information.

National Center for Education in Maternal & Child Health, (202) 784-9770. Offers information on pregnancy, maternity, and genetic inherited disorders that may affect the whole family. Mailing address: Georgetown University, Box 571272, Washington, DC 20057. Web site: www.ncemch.org. No Spanish on Web site.

National Child Support Enforcement Association, tel. (202) 624-8180, fax (202) 624-8828. Nonprofit membership organization representing the child support community, a workforce of over 60,000. Their mission is to promote the well-being of children through professional development of its membership advocacy and public awareness. Address: 444 North Capitol St., Suite 414, Washington, DC 20001-1512. Web site: www.ncsea.org.

The National Department of Health and Human Services of the United States, (800) 336-4797. Referral number where you can get information on prenatal care and other social services. To get a brochure, you may call directly (202) 619-0257. Or you may request a free brochure called "Prenatal Care"(OHDS 73-30017), which offers mothers basic information about pregnancy and caring for a newborn baby. Request it by mentioning the above title and number and writing to: DEPARTMENT OF HEALTH AND HUMAN SERVICES Office of Human Development Services, LSDS, Department 76, Washington, DC 20401. www.hhs.gov/ (English); www.healthfinder.gov/español/ (Spanish).

National Maternal & Child Health Clearing House, (888) ASK-HRSA (275-4772). Offers a free *Health Diary,* with useful information for the expectant mother. The book is available in English and Spanish. They also have lists of books and articles related to pregnancy and child care. Web site: www.ask.hrsa.gov/. Information in Spanish on Web site.

National Organization of Mothers of Twins Club, (505) 275-0955. Encompasses more than 300 clubs created by mothers who have had multiple births. They offer information and advice. Address: P.O. Box 700860, Plymouth, MI 48170-0955. Web site: www.nomotc.org. Spanish on Web site. E-mail: info@nomotc.ogr.

National Organization of Single Mothers, Inc. (NOSM), (704) 888-KIDS. Clearinghouse of information and network of support to single mothers. Helps establish support groups and publishes a bimonthly newsletter Address: SingleMOTHER, PO Box 68, Midland, NC 28107. Web site: http://singlemothers.org.

National Organization of Working Women, (800) 522-0925. Open from 9AM to 5PM, they offer guidance on labor rights for pregnant mothers and new mothers on the job. Free informational brochures are available in Spanish. Address: 1430 W Peachtree St., # 610, Atlanta, GA 30309. Web site: www.9to5.org.

National Resource Center for Parents with Disabilities, (800) 644-2666 or (510) 848-1112. Web site: www.lookingglass.org. Spanish on Web site.

National STD Hotline. AIDS and sexually transmitted disease confidential information. Web site: www.ashastd.org/nah. (800) 243-7889; (800) 227-8922; or (800) 342-2437. Open 24 hours a day, 7 days a week.

National Women's Health Information Center (NWHIC), (800) 994-WOMAN (9662). Provides information on women's health and breast-feeding. (English and Spanish.)

National Women's Health Organization, (202) 347-1140. Provides information on women's health and guidance in the event of litigation related to the subject. Address: 514 10th St. NW, Suite 400, Washington, DC 20005.

Newborn Hearing Screening Program (California), (877) 388-5301 (English and Spanish). Hearing tests for newborns. Web site: www.dhs.ca.gov/pcfh/cms/nhsp/.

Pacific Post-Partum Support Society. Address: 104-1416 Commercial Dr., Vancouver, BC V5L3X9. (604) 255-7999 (Canadian number). Web site: www.postpartum.org. No Spanish on Web site.

Planned Parenthood, www.plannedparenthood.org/ (English); www.plannedparenthood.org/espanol (Spanish).

Post-Partum Education for Parents (PEP), (805) 564-3888. Offers emotional support to mothers, administered by volunteer parents, as well as basic education on infant care and the role of new parents. They have several publications in English and Spanish. Address: PO Box 6154, Santa Barbara, CA 93110. Web site: www.sbpep.org.

Pregnancy Hotline, (800) 395-HELP. Information for pregnant teenagers on where they can receive medical and social services. Web site: www.pregnancycenters.org.

Pregnancy and Parental Leave Resource Kit. A booklet that explains the Family and Medical Leave Act in greater detail. The cost is $5. Address: The NOW Legal Defense and Education Fund, 99 Hudson St., New York, NY 10013.

Pregnancy Risk Hotline, (801) 323-2229. Offers free brochures to persons in Utah and Montana (state funds), as well as information to persons in other states regarding similar organizations in their area. They provide information on the risks caused by chemical products, drugs, medication, and toxic infections during pregnancy. They offer translation services in 37 languages, including Spanish.

Pregnancy Today, www.pregnancytoday.com. No Spanish on Web site. English journal with articles (in Spanish, *Embarazo Hoy*). iParenting.com, PO Box 1780, Evanston IL 60204. E-mail: info@iparenting.com. (847) 556-2300; (800) 444-0064 (toll-free).

Resolve, (301) 652-8585 or (888) 623-0744 (toll-free) English/Spanish. The National Infertility Association. Emotional support and medical references for couples who have been unable to conceive. Address: 7910 Woodmont Avenue, Suite 1350, Bethesda, MD 20814. Web site: www.resolve.org.

Ser Padres magazine, (800) 982-1564 (for subscriptions). A Spanish-language version of *Parents'* magazine. The most up-to-date information on pregnancy education, baby health, and family nutrition, Six issues a year for $6.

Single Mothers by Choice, (704) 888-KIDS. Clearinghouse of information and network of support to single mothers. Helps establish support groups and publishes a bimonthly newsletter. Address: SingleMOTHER, PO Box 68, Midland, NC 28107. Web site: www.solomother@aol.comhttp://singlemothers.org.

Triplet Connection, (435) 851-1105. Offers support and advice to mothers with triplets or more, as well as information on how to avoid premature delivery. Address: PO Box 429, Spring City, UT 84662. Web site: www.tripletconnection.org. No Spanish on Web site.

TWINS magazine, www.twinsmagazine.com. (888) 55-TWINS (Subscription order line).The Internet magazine for parents of twins, with additional links to other resources for parents of multiples. English.

U.S. Directory of Health and Human Services Data Resources, www.aspe.os.dhhs.gov/_/index.cfm. English.

WIC (Women, Infants, and Children). Web site: www.fns.usda.gov/wic/Contacts/tollfreenumbers.htm; www.fns.usda.gov/wic/Contacts/statealpha.htm. Toll-free numbers are different for each state: (888) WIC-WORKS (942-9675) (CA); (800) 533-5006 (NY). English and Spanish. This organization safeguards the health of low-income women, infants, and children up to age five who are at risk due to poor nutrition. They provide nutritious foods and dietary supplements according to their health status and their needs. They also provide information on healthy eating and referrals to health care. Web site: www.fns.usda.gov/wic/.

Women's Bureau Publications. Request a summary of the laws in your state regarding maternity leave. Address: U.S. Department of Labor, Box EX, 200 Constitution Avenue NW, Washington, DC 20210.

Zero to Three, www.zerotothree.org. Early child development Web site for parents and professionals.

WEB SITES FOR FAMILY-RELATED ISSUES
Family Planet: www.family.starware.com/
Family.com: www.family.com/
Parent Soup: www.parentsoup.com/
ParentTime: www.pathfinder.com/ParentTime/
Family Education Network: www.families.com/

GLOSSARY

A brief dictionary for the expectant mother

A

Abortion: Termination of a pregnancy before the end of the twentieth week. It can be spontaneous or induced.

Acupuncture: Procedure that consists of placing needles under the skin in specific areas of the human body, to relieve pain and help combat certain addictions (smoking, for example).

Additives: Substances included in most processed foods, some of which may be harmful. The most common are food coloring, sweeteners, artificial flavors, caffeine, and monosodium glutamate.

Adrenaline: Hormone secreted by the adrenal glands. Adrenaline accelerates heart rate, increases blood pressure, dilates the bronchi, and affects digestion.

AIDS: A deficiency of the immune (defense) system due to infection with the human immunodeficiency virus (HIV), AIDS (acquired immune deficiency syndrome) can remain quiet, without causing symptoms, for long periods of time, or it can cause symptoms because of the inability of the infected person's body to fight infections and cancer. It is diagnosed from a blood test for antibodies that the body produces to fight it. The virus is spread most often by sexual contact but may be spread by contaminated blood or needles. The mother can infect the fetus during pregnancy.

Alpha-fetoprotein: Substance produced by the fetus and found in the amniotic fluid and the blood of the mother. Elevated levels suggest the possibility of defects in the spinal cord (nervous system) of the fetus.

Amino acids: Substances that serve as building blocks for protein.

Amniocentesis: The extraction of amniotic fluid for analysis.

Anemia: Low red blood cell count.

Anencephaly: Absence at birth of the brain, top of the skull, and spinal cord. It may be detected by a test that measures the level of alpha-fetoprotein in the amniotic fluid or the mother's blood.

B

Biopsy: Microscopic examination of tissue for diagnostic purposes.

Blood types: There are four blood types: O, A, B, and AB. When someone receives a blood transfusion, it must be of the same type so that the antibodies in the donated blood don't react against the recipient's blood.

Braxton-Hicks contractions: Irregular contractions of the uterus that occur during pregnancy.

C

Calorie: Unit of nutrition measurement: The energy value or nutritional power of foods is determined by calories. If a pregnant woman's physical activity is light, she must multiply her ideal weight by twelve; by fifteen if her activity is moderate, and by twenty if she is very active. She should then add 300 to 500 to the number obtained; and the result is her daily requirement of calories during pregnancy.

Carbohydrates: Nutritional substances that provide energy. Divided into starches and sugars. The complex carbohydrates are found in whole grain cereals, vegetables, and fruits. The simple carbohydrates and sugars are a quick source of energy that do not contribute to the baby's growth, so should preferably be substituted by fruits that also provide vitamins, minerals, and fiber.

Chlamydia: Sexually transmitted disease that may infect the urethra, anus, or female organs, causing inflammation of the pelvis. When symptoms are present, they may include painful intercourse, frequent urination with a burning sensation, and stomach pain. Erythromycin is the most frequently prescribed medication for pregnant women suffering from chlamydia, to avoid infecting the baby during delivery.

Chorionic membrane: Placenta tissue. Analyzing it during pregnancy allows evaluation of the condition of the fetus.

Chorionic tissue test: Diagnostic study that analyzes placental tissue in the early stages of pregnancy to evaluate certain fetal abnormalities.

Chromosome: Element of the nucleus of the cells. The number of chromosomes is always constant in each and every cell of an individual, and in all individuals of the same species.

Circumcision: Minor surgery consisting of a circular incision on the foreskin (loose skin that covers the head of the male genital). Generally practiced on baby boys a few days after birth to prevent infections, which may also be prevented by bathing them regularly and pulling the foreskin back to avoid accumulation of dirt or soap residue.

Cleft lip: Congenital vertical split in the upper lip. It may be partial or extend all the way to the base of the nose, and it may be on one or both sides of the nose.

Cleft palate: Congenital gap along the roof of the mouth. It runs the length of the middle of the palate, extending from behind the teeth to the cavity of the nose. Sometimes it is an extension of a cleft lip.

Colostrum: First milk that the mother secretes at the end of her pregnancy. It is a yellowish, watery fluid that changes in composition after delivery.

Conjunctivitis: Inflammation of the inner membrane of the eyelids and front of the eye.

Cystitis: Infection of the bladder, frequently due to an infection.

D

Diabetes: Elevated blood sugar (glucose) levels. When it develops during pregnancy, it is known as gestational diabetes.

Dyspnea: Difficulty breathing.

E

Eclampsia or toxemia: Convulsions and coma in patient with preeclampsia (see preeclampsia).

Ectopic pregnancy: Pregnancy that occurs outside the uterine cavity, for example, in one of the fallopian tubes (that connect the ovaries to the uterus).

Endometriosis: Proliferation of the tissue that covers the womb (endometrium) outside the uterine cavity.

Episiotomy: Surgical incision at the opening of the vagina made during delivery to avoid lacerations and tearing in that area.

Essential amino acids: Eight amino acids that the body cannot produce and must be retrieved from foods.

Estrogen: Female hormone produced by the ovaries during the woman's reproductive age.

F

Fallopian tubes: Parts of the female reproductive system that carry the ovum to the uterus.

Fetal suffering: Problems in the fetus that occur before birth or during labor and require an immediate delivery.

Fibroma: Benign fibrous tumor in the uterus.

Folic acid: One of the B-complex vitamins. Very important to the growth of cells, especially during pregnancy. Daily recommended dosage for pregnant women is one milligram. Reduces the risk of defects in the baby's nervous system.

G

Gene: Each of the elements that are arranged in linear and fixed manner the length of the chromosomes and that determine hereditary characteristics.

Genital herpes: Sexually transmitted disease produced by a virus that provokes painful blisters in the genital area. When present during delivery a cesarean section may be indicated to prevent transmission to the baby.

Gestation: Pregnancy.

Gingivitis: Inflammation of the gums.

Globulin: Blood component involved in coagulation.

Gonorrhea: Sexually transmitted disease caused by a bacteria known as gonococcus. Can be treated with antibiotics. If the woman is suffering from gonorrhea during delivery, her baby may be blinded at birth.

Gynecology: Study of female-related diseases.

H

Hemophilia: An inherited bleeding disorder characterized by recurrent bleeding. It is caused by a deficiency of a specific blood protein.

High-risk pregnancy: Problems and complications during pregnancy that may signal the need to see a specialist.

Hyperglycemia: Elevated blood sugar (glucose).

Hypermesis gravidarum: Severe nausea and vomiting during pregnancy that can cause dehydration and may require hospitalization for treatment. Generally in the first trimester.

Hypertension: High blood pressure.

Hypotension: Abnormally low blood pressure.

I

Immune: Not susceptible to certain diseases. A mother who has Rh-negative factor and whose child is Rh positive is vaccinated with immune globulin of her Rh type, to avoid harm to future pregnancies.

IUD: Intrauterine device. Placed inside the uterus, it functions as a contraceptive; in other words, it prevents unwanted pregnancies by avoiding implantation of the egg in the uterine wall.

L

Labor: Rhythmic contractions that cause the cervix to dilate and allow the baby to emerge.

Laparoscopy: Surgery that allows examination of the abdomen using a laparoscope. This instrument goes through the abdominal wall by way of small perforations made by the surgeon.

Late-term baby: Pregnancy that lasts more than forty-two weeks.

Lochia: Vaginal discharge in the weeks following delivery. It can last up to six weeks.

M

Meconium: The first feces of the fetus.

Morning sickness: Nausea and vomiting that occur especially in the first trimester.

Muscular dystrophy: An inherited muscle disorder of unknown cause in which there is slow but progressive degeneration of muscle fibers.

N

Natural childbirth: Labor and delivery without painkillers.

O

Obstetrics: Branch of medicine that studies gestation, delivery, and puerperium.

Organic fluids: Liquids of the body.

Ovulation: Release of the ovum within the ovary in women with regular menstrual periods, this happens during the time between the ten days following the previous menstruation and the ten days before the following menstruation. In other words, an eight-day time frame.

Ovum (plural: ova): Female sexual cell which, fertilized, originates the embryo.

Oxytocin: Hormone produced by the body during labor, delivery, and puerperium. Also given to induce labor since it causes the uterus to contract.

P

Pelvis: Body cavity located in the lower part of the abdomen. It contains the reproductive organs, fallopian tubes, and the uterus.

Pharmacopeia: Medicinal substances and their combinations.

Placenta: The only organ that connects the fetus to the mother by means of the umbilical cord. It is attached to the inside of the womb. Its function is to feed the fetus during pregnancy.

Preeclampsia: Development of high blood pressure, fluid retention, swelling, and protein in the urine, toward the end of pregnancy.

Premature delivery: Delivery before week thirty-eight of pregnancy.

Progesterone: Female sexual hormone secreted in large quantities during the gestation period. For this reason it is known as the "pregnancy hormone."

Proteins: Substances that function as the building material for the tissues of the body. Proteins are vital to the developing fetus. It is recommended that a pregnant woman ingest 70 to 80 grams of protein daily.

Puerperium: Period following delivery until the uterus returns to normal size.

Pyorrhea: Gum disease that can cause the loosening and eventual loss of teeth.

R

Reproductive organs: Organs in charge of reproduction. In the female, her ovaries; in the male, his testicles.

Rupture of the amniotic membranes: Also called breaking of the water. The amniotic sac breaks releasing the amniotic fluid.

S

Somatic problems: Problems concerning the body.

Spina bifida: Open spine, a congenital defect of the spinal cord in which part of one (or more) vertebrae fail to develop completely, leaving a section of the spinal cord exposed. It may be detected by means of the alpha-fetoprotein test.

T

Tar: Dark, resinous substance obtained by distilling coal or pine wood. Present in the paper used in producing cigarettes.

Thyroid: Gland, located in front of the trachea, which produces a hormone, thyroxin, which is involved in growth and metabolism.

U

Umbilical cord: Cord that connects the fetus at its navel to the placenta (the organ inside the mother's uterus). It permits the transport of nutritive elements and oxygen from the mother to the fetus and the elimination of waste and carbon dioxide from the fetus to the mother through the placenta.

Uterus: Womb.

V

Vaginal plug: Mucous plug formed from secretions of the cervix; it comes out close to the time of delivery or during labor.

Vaginitis: Inflammation of the vagina, usually due to an infection.

Venereal: That which is transmitted by sexual contact.

Vitamins: Substances that exist in foods and that are necessary to the balance of all the functions of the body.

> *Vitamin A:* Necessary for growth and repair of cellular membranes, it helps maintain the health of the external part of the skin as well as the lining of the stomach, the intestines, the respiratory system, and the liver. Also related to eye health.
>
> *B vitamins:* Necessary during pregnancy for the growth of the fetus. Their deficiency is related to blood disorders and mental retardation.
>
> *Vitamin C:* Needed so the cell wall and the blood vessels are strong; also helps control some pregnancy discomforts such as softening of the gums and nosebleeds.
>
> *Vitamin D:* Regulates the absorption of calcium.
>
> *Vitamin E:* Helps normal growth of the fetus.
>
> *Vitamin K:* Indispensable for blood coagulation.

INDEX

abdomen
 changes in, 119
 pain in, 20, 107, 203
 shape of, myth concerning, 14
abortions, 26–28
 ethical considerations concerning, 26–27
 health considerations concerning, 27–28
 previous, 36–37
 statistics concerning illegal, 28
abruptio placenta, 122
AIDS. *See* HIV/AIDS
Alan Gutmacher Institute of New York
 illegal abortions report, 28
alcohol abuse, 66–67
allergies, 120
alpha-fetoprotein, prenatal testing for, 65–66
American Medical Association
 caffeine report, 71
 position on abortion, 27
amniocentesis, 19, 45, 62–63
 indications for, 63
analgesics, 189
anemia, 58, 119–120
anencephaly, 66
anesthesia, 189–190
 general, 190
 regional nerve block, 189–190
 types of, 189
Answer One-Step home pregnancy test, 12
Apgar index, 197
asthma, 113

back pain, 106–107
birth, 9, 81
 baby's arrival, 187
 in delivery room, 185–188
 first minutes after, 188

pushing and contractions during, 186
 pushing positions during, 186
birth control, 27
 after forty, 44
 first diaphragm, 216
 postpartum, 215
birth rates, ranked by month, 175
Birth Without Violence (Leboyer), 129
birthing classes, 127
 exercises, 128
 Lamaze method, 128–129
 Leboyer method, 129
 objectives and benefits of, 127
birthmarks, myth concerning, 129
births
 Latin America's record for, 46
 world's record for, 46
bladder infections, 115
blood incompatibility (Rh factor), 36–37,
 43–44, 62
blood pressure, high, 114
 medicines, 70
body aches, postpartum, 203
body changes
 abdominal, 119
 breasts, 118–119
bones and joints, aching, 107
bottle feeding, 212–213
Braxton Hicks contractions, 105
breast-feeding
 advantages of, 208–209
 diet during, 211
 learning, 210–211
 statistics concerning, 208
 your wardrobe during, 212
breasts
 changes in, 118–119
 swollen, postpartum, 205

ALIZA A. LIFSHITZ, M.D., is well known to the Hispanic community and has been its primary source of trusted health information, appearing as a health reporter for the Univision TV Network since 1988. In addition to her practice, she currently reports on *Primer Impacto*, Spanish-language television's highest rated news magazine, and is the face of Univision's Health Initiative, *Entérate*. Her call-in program, *El Consultorio de la Dra. Aliza*, airs weekly on the Univision Radio network. Dr. Aliza's weekly column in *La Opinión* is syndicated in newspapers throughout the country. She is also executive publisher of *Prevention En Español* magazine. She is four-time president of the California Hispanic-American Medical Association and was selected by the American Medical Association to launch its 1992 Medical Ethics Consumer Information Campaign.